T0336217

THE THIRD NET

The Third Net

The Hidden System of
Migrant Health Care

Lisa Sun-Hee Park,
Erin Hoekstra, *and*
Anthony M. Jimenez

NEW YORK UNIVERSITY PRESS
New York

NEW YORK UNIVERSITY PRESS
New York
www.nyupress.org

© 2024 by New York University
All rights reserved

Please contact the Library of Congress for Cataloging-in-Publication data.

ISBN: 9781479821556 (hardback)
ISBN: 9781479821563 (paperback)
ISBN: 9781479821594 (library ebook)
ISBN: 9781479821570 (consumer ebook)

This book is printed on acid-free paper, and its binding materials are chosen for strength and durability. We strive to use environmentally responsible suppliers and materials to the greatest extent possible in publishing our books.

Manufactured in the United States of America

10 9 8 7 6 5 4 3 2 1

Also available as an ebook

To all those working toward health justice in the Third Net.

CONTENTS

Introduction

Infrastructure of the Third Net

Like most clinics of its kind, it has no distinguishing marks to signal its internal workings. The small, nondescript, rectangular, single-story building is covered in varying shades of brown and beige paint after so many years of neglect. There are no signs to indicate that this is a medical facility that fulfills a crucial role in the overall health care system. The entry doorway opens to two waiting rooms. On the left, people are quietly sitting, and on the right, volunteer nurses, doctors, and medical students are briskly walking in and out of a series of small examination rooms that snake all the way to the back door. A handwritten sign on the wall reads: "We only and exclusively give care to undocumented people."

The clinic opens at 6 or 6:30 am most mornings and there is always a line. There are no appointments. People must arrive early and wait, and even then, there is no guarantee that they will be seen by the two doctors—both formally retired from their profession years ago. The wait for the dentist is even longer since she only visits once or twice a month, and there is a raffle system to decide who will get to see her today. A friendly woman with an easy smile, the dentist admits that all she can really do at the clinic is pull teeth, but that does not stop the local hospital from referring uninsured migrant patients to her. In the next room is an endocrinologist who focuses almost exclusively on diabetic patients. A migrant from South America, he has been retired for years but continues to volunteer at the clinic two days a week. This is what health care looks like for undocumented migrants in the United States—if they are lucky. This is the Third Net.

* * *

Underneath the formal safety net system of health care is an informal, threadbare, and disconnected assortment of organizations that provide basic care to millions of migrants across the country. With wildly vary-ing levels of service, organizational culture, and mission, a patchwork of free, or nearly free, health care exists for those excluded from the formal health system. There are mobile clinics rotating from one church parking lot to another, one Saturday a month. Another clinic is a "pop-up"—temporarily repurposing an office building after hours, with their files and supplies stashed in a closet until their weekly use. Yet another is a nondescript little house, once abandoned for years, refurbished into a makeshift, unlicensed clinic run by health activists. What is consistent, however, is that there is always a line of people quietly waiting, despite no visible sign or welcoming marquee. A passerby who did not already know what it was would never know.

The central contribution of this book is to document the existence of a Third Net and to provide a glimpse into these spaces and what they tell us about the larger vulnerabilities of the structure of the health care safety net in the United States. More specifically, we investigate the health care safety net for undocumented, low-income, and uninsured migrants in the United States. In focusing on one of the most marginal-ized communities, we approach the jumble of health care providers that form a patchwork safety net across the country as an *infrastructure* that is hierarchically organized in distinct but interactive levels, or nets. In this way, we outline the logic that orders the *purposive disarray of care*. The population at the center of our study resides in the Third Net of a larger safety net system—of public hospitals, community health centers, federally qualified health centers, and non-governmental organizations whose mission is to provide care to people regardless of ability to pay.[1]

In approaching the Third Net as an infrastructure, we analyze the or-ganizational structure and the discourses and social interactions within each clinic to illustrate the variety and contradictions across multiple re-gions. At the same time, we observe how these individual organizations actually operate collectively in support of a larger system of US health care.[2] This approach helped us to not only understand the mechanisms of each organization but also how these seemingly disparate, discon-nected, and wide-ranging clinics and organizations combined to form the basis of a larger societal project.

Our study found that the informal infrastructure of the Third Net buttressed the formal system by serving as a "dumping ground" for the formal health care system. The Third Net absorbs the inefficiencies, illogic, and cruelty of modern poverty governance, as exemplified by the formal health care system. And, as the subsequent chapters will show, the Third Net develops its own set of infrastructural networks and attendant logics to manage and organize the systemic messiness with which it must contend. The multiple methods used in our study allowed us to grasp both the granular details of an organization and its overarching role within a not-always-apparent structure. We began with an exploratory pilot study in which we visited safety net hospitals, clinics, local migrant health advocates, and key regional health policy administrators in cities within the four US states that border Mexico: Texas, New Mexico, Arizona, and California. Our initial objective was to document the impact of the newly implemented Patient Protection and Affordable Care Act (ACA) on undocumented migrants. As we began to understand how the states varied in their larger history and politics toward migrants, we decided to focus primarily on Texas and Arizona for a deeper exploration of undocumented health care access. This book will highlight the interviews and ethnographies we conducted of the Third Net in Houston, Texas, and Phoenix and Tucson, Arizona. Key respondents who were directly engaged in safety net health care provision offered important vantage points from each region, and we quickly became aware that we needed to better comprehend the social structure underlying the impact of this major federal policy. It also became clear that low-income migrants' access to the health care safety net was an important route to do so. Subsequently, we conducted year-long ethnographies within Third Net health care organizations in Arizona and Texas to discern, in detail, the infrastructure within a particular region and its connection to the overall Third Net.

US Migrant Health Care

Health care for migrants remains a politically volatile issue.[3] Currently, even those that fit the ideal of a "good" migrant—hard-working, silent, invisible, and able-bodied—are considered undeserving of health care due to their noncitizen status and racialization. Demographic transformation in the United States has precipitated intense political debates regarding the social and economic costs and benefits of immigration

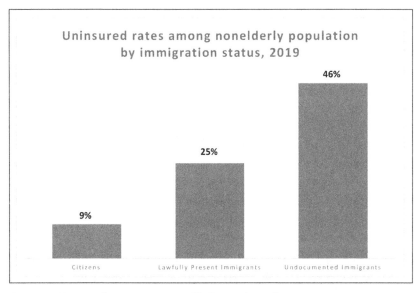

Figure I.1. Uninsured rates among nonelderly population by immigration status, 2019. Source: Kaiser Family Foundation Analysis of 2019 American Community Survey, 1-year estimates, cited in Samantha Artiga, Nambi Ndugga, and Olivia Pham, "Immigrant Access to COVID-19 Vaccines: Key Issues to Consider," Henry J. Kaiser Family Foundation, January 13, 2021, www.kff.org.

and migrants, the majority of whom are from Latin America and Asia.[4] One of the most passionately argued reasons against immigration is the use of health care by those who are undocumented and the alleged related costs of uncompensated care on public hospitals and community health centers.

Since 1970, immigration has increased significantly, and as of 2019, there were 22.5 million noncitizens[5] and 22.9 million naturalized citizens residing in the US, making up 14% of the total population. Of the noncitizen population, 11 million are estimated to be undocumented.[6] Among the nonelderly[7] population in 2019, undocumented migrants had the highest rate of uninsurance (see figure I.1).[8] The differences based on citizenship/immigration status are stark: 46% of undocumented migrants were uninsured, compared to 25% of documented migrants and 8% of citizens.[9]

With the implementation of the Affordable Care Act, undocumented migrants have disappeared as a patient population from the formal safety net. In fact, an important factor in the passage of the ACA, the most significant federal health care legislation since the creation of Medicaid and Medicare in 1965, was the explicit exclusion of undocumented migrants from its provisions. The contentiousness of this issue was evident on September 9, 2009, when Representative Joe Wilson of South Carolina interrupted President Obama during his speech to Congress presenting his new health care reform plan and shrieked, "You lie!" This unprecedented outburst occurred when the president spoke specifically to the issue of undocumented migrants' continued denial of health care access. As a *New York Times* editorial later stated, "Illegal immigration is an all-purpose policy explosive."[10] At the time of its passage, the Affordable Care Act was the largest expansion of social policy in the US in a generation.[11] Arguably the most consequential and controversial social policy enacted in years, with wide-ranging impacts on nearly every aspect of the health care infrastructure, the ACA was also the signature policy of President Barack Obama.[12] The fact that this major reform was passed under the first black president contributed to the political contentiousness of this legislation. A number of studies found that racial attitudes were highly correlated with support for the ACA.[13]

A baffling aspect of this volatile politics of migrant health care access is that undocumented migrants and newly arrived documented migrants (including legal permanent residents who have been in the US for less than five years) were ineligible for publicly funded health insurance before the ACA and continued to remain ineligible under President Obama's new plan. Technically speaking, there is no difference with respect to undocumented migrant health care access. And yet, this issue continues not only to enrage but also to drive public sentiment and public policy. "The immigrant" appears to trigger a fundamental national anxiety regarding access to essential public goods such as health care, and the stridently hostile politics of deservingness and social belonging associated with migrant health care show little sign of abating.

Consequently, the exclusion of undocumented migrants was directly tied to the expansion of Medicaid to millions of low-income citizens. The rights of citizens were framed as mutually exclusive and in opposition to the rights of migrants. And while this does not mark a drastic change in prior eligibility requirements for undocumented migrants, its provisions to insure greater numbers of citizens coincide with safety net hospitals restructuring their services to cater to these newly insured patients and a decrease in federal funding to cover the costs of uncompensated care. As a result, the formal health care safety net for uninsured migrants has significantly diminished in size and scope.[14] These changes, coupled with restrictive immigration policy, have significantly limited the health care access of this population and heightened the importance of an informal Third Net of care.

The US Health System and Its Safety Nets

There is no single system of health care in the United States. Instead, it is a complex mix of private and public, for-profit and nonprofit, insurers and health care providers. The following figure from the Commonwealth Fund is useful in graphically outlining the overall health care system in the US:[15]

Perhaps the most notable feature of this figure is the central role of financing in organizing the system. While interconnected to some extent, US health care is separated into public and private payer systems. All the arrows move downward, from the initial funding source to the various complexities of regulatory organizations, health-related institutions and centers, and end with the providers (and pharmacies).

As of 2018, 67.3% of the population had some form of private health insurance and 34.4% had public insurance.[16] The vast majority of private insurance was purchased through an employer and the remainder purchased directly.[17] Those with public insurance are overwhelmingly covered through Medicare or Medicaid. The federally funded Medicare program covers adults age 65 and older and some people with disabilities, Medicaid covers people with low income, and the Children's Health Insurance Program (CHIP) provides low-cost coverage for children in families that earn too much to qualify for Medicaid. An additional 1% of insurance coverage is federally funded by the military and Department of Veterans Affairs.

These publicly financed programs, whether supported by federal, state, and/or local government funds, constitute the formal safety net. Public hospitals, community clinics, and Federally Qualified Health Centers (FQHCs)[18] provide the bulk of the primary and preventative care for those with low income and without insurance. In addition, a federal law that

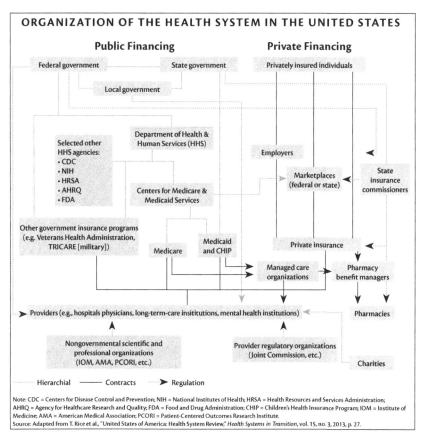

Figure I.2. Organization of the health system in the United States. Source: T. Rice et al., "United States of America: Health System Review," *Health Systems in Transition* 15, no. 3 (2013), p. 27.

requires most hospitals to provide emergency care regardless of ability to pay or insurance status allows some level of access to private hospitals as well. In return, Medicare and Medicaid provide "disproportionate-share payments" to hospitals with large numbers of patients who are publicly insured or uninsured to offset the uncompensated care costs. Local and state taxes also contribute toward charity care and safety net health programs through public hospitals and local health departments.

In general, the quality of care by the publicly financed safety net is viewed as secondary or inferior to the quality of a private hospital or

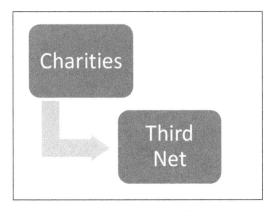

Figure I.3. Organization of the Third Net

program, and the patients in the safety net are commonly viewed as those excluded from the private payer insurance program. The terminology used in describing the safety net assumes that an individual "falls" through the gaps of a superior quality of care and lands on a lesser level of health care providers. The infrastructure of the safety net, with its cobbling together of financing across a complex web of federal, state, and local contributions, and wide variations in type and quality of care from one region to another, contributes to its reputation as an unstable and lesser form of health care for those without better options.

However uneven, this overall system of private and public health insurance options encompasses 91.5% of the US population. The remaining 8.5% are uninsured—a significant decrease from 16% in 2010, the year in which the ACA became law.[19] The Third Net exists within this marginal, informal space.

Disconnected from the standard financial infrastructure, the Third Net is located in a parallel context, a fuzzy shadow that extends past the existing arrows in the complex figure above. A map of the Third Net begins with the "charity" box located in the far lower-right corner of figure I.2, with an arrow extending to another page, showing what appears to be a far simpler infrastructure. Without direct connection to formal public or private financing, the Third Net is invisible, and its "chart" might look something like what appears in figure I.3.

However, our research delves into this neglected sector and maps a different, far more intricate system within a system. The Third Net has an infrastructure of its own, driven by a network of interpersonal relationships and informal funding sources. As informal providers, organizations within the Third Net may not be regulated by the state or even acknowledged as health care entities by government agencies. They comprise free clinics and small community-based organizations that provide limited primary care or simply preventative care. Most, if not all, of their funding comes from private sources in the form of charitable giving, and labor is largely voluntary and without pay.

While it is located outside the formal health care system, including the formal first and second tiers of the safety net, the Third Net is intricately connected to the overall health care system. The organizations and volunteers in the Third Net attend to those whom the formal system is unable or unwilling to serve. Consequently, policy changes to the First and Second Nets reverberate to the Third.

The First Net of the health care safety net is composed mostly of large and medium-sized hospitals that treat a significant proportion of the state's Medicaid or uninsured population (see table 1).[20] These hospitals, generally located in large metropolitan areas, serve as anchors of the formal health care safety net system. They provide a wide range of health services—including primary, specialist, and emergency care—and their funding is largely dependent on government funds. The Second Net is a network of community health clinics including FQHCs. Some of these community health clinics may be offshoots of larger public hospitals (i.e., First Net). They provide limited health services for low-income, uninsured, and underinsured people on a sliding scale and are dependent

TABLE 1.1. Safety nets of health care

Safety Net	Formal/ Informal	Type of Facility	Type of Care	Primary Funding
First Net	Formal	Hospitals	Primary Specialist Emergency	Government (public)
Second Net	Formal	Community health clinics Federally qualified health centers	Primary Ad hoc specialist Preventative	Government (public)
Third Net	Informal	Free clinics Nonprofit community organizations	Limited primary Preventative	Charity (private)

primarily upon government funding. The Third Net extends the safety net beyond the formal health care system to serve those with nowhere else to go and without the funds to pay for care in the other nets.

The Third Net's informality within the health care safety net serves important medical, economic, and political functions. Its liminal position as not entirely underground but not fully acknowledged as a health care provider allows Third Net organizations to serve marginalized populations without being hindered by some of the more punitive surveillance requirements. For instance, because they do not accept federal Medicaid funds, these organizations are not subject to government requirements to ask patients their citizenship status. However, this also means Third Net organizations have limited funds and the range of medical care offered is severely constrained. Economically, the Third Net functions as a form of charity care and, like charity in general, raises a number of concerns regarding its role in reinforcing a system of inequality. Certainly, there is concern that the Third Net is too convenient a dumping ground for the uninsured by the formal safety net. Politically, the concentration of this population into this informal sector reinforces the perception of low-income undocumented migrants as outsiders and undeserving of social services. This community becomes segregated into a nonviable patient population and beyond the formal safety net's area of concern. Consequently, the existence of the Third Net, which is the result of an unequal infrastructure, can also function to maintain the unjust system.

From the vantage point of the Third Net, the US health system is organized in a rigid hierarchy, with the Third Net relegated to the bottom and yet upholding the system overall (see figure I.4).[21] At the top of the inverted pyramid is the for-profit health care sector, which is geared to those with private health insurance. It is formally structured with paid employees and multiple sources of financing, much of it private. Below this is the safety net, which is further divided into multiple layers of care, for low-income individuals who are underinsured or uninsured.

As its name suggests, the safety net is a loosely configured web of organizations stretched to catch those who fall outside the private health insurance market.[22] It is commonly and appropriately described as a "patchwork" of insecure and irregular services that vary greatly from

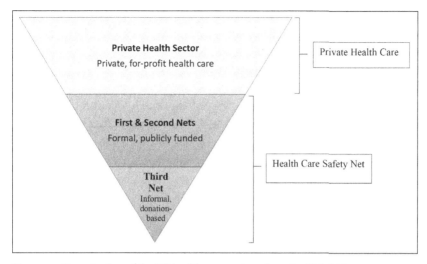

Figure 1.4. Organization of the US health care system, from the Third Net

one town, city, county, or state to another. The public hospitals of the First Net and the community health clinics of the Second Net are considered "core" safety nets. Many facilities in the First Net provide critical specialized services such as trauma care, burn care, and neonatal care in some urban regions and train large numbers of physicians and other health professionals. The First and Second Net organizations are formally structured and heavily bureaucratized, with paid employees and a budget that is largely publicly funded. Its financing structure is also restrictive in how they cover their costs. While non–safety net, or private, providers have the ability to shift the cost of uncompensated care onto other private insurance revenues, core safety net providers rely on public sources of funds such as Medicaid, which are restricted from reallocating these costs from one patient population to another. Core safety nets are also dependent on federally set rates of compensation that many times do not adequately cover the actual cost of health care.[23] However, despite these constraints, studies have documented quality care by core safety net organizations that meets or exceeds private health care.[24]

Beneath this First and Second Net lies the Third Net. It is distinctive in its informal organizational structure, lack of paid employees, and donation funding base. A number of organizations in the Third Net are not just nonprofit but nonexistent as a source of health care, meaning some organizations are not acknowledged as a health care provider at all. In every way, the Third Net appears misplaced and anachronistic as part of this system. And yet, as we will show, it is pivotal to the function of the overall infrastructure precisely because of its unique features. For instance, as mentioned earlier, core safety net hospitals have limited and restricted revenue sources in comparison to private hospitals and must adhere to complex governance and leadership structures that accompany public funds. Ironically, as marginalized entities with little to no government funds, Third Net organizations operate unencumbered by these restrictions. Of course, there are significant and obvious downsides to relying on individual charity—the kinds of care provided and the number of patients seen are severely limited, and the infrastructural foundations are highly unstable in comparison to other formally recognized safety net organizations. Also, freedom from governmental restrictions does not mean they do not have any rules. In fact, we show how organizations in the Third Net take great pains to develop their own guidelines and mission, and they collectively contribute toward an infrastructure across states and regions that allow for the functionality of the overall health system.

In other words, the infrastructural instability of the informal performs an important function in the stability of the formal. The so-called patchwork has a logic of its own and serves a larger purpose. It is no coincidence that Third Net organizations regularly receive patients referred to them by hospitals and clinics in the private sector and the two core safety nets. The Third Net becomes a convenient location to push out patients for whom there are no routes for compensation for their care, even for safety net providers whose mission is to care for those with low income and no insurance. This is particularly the case for safety net providers living in states that did not expand Medicaid under the Affordable Care Act. And, just as importantly, the Third Net absorbs the messiness and cruelties of the overall health care system. It is used to hide the realities of an exclusionary system that discriminates on the basis of class, race, and immigration status. It is from this broader, infrastructural framing that we began to understand these referrals as a form of patient dumping.

Patient Dumping from One Net to Another

"Patient dumping" generally refers to the transfer of a patient from a private to a public hospital for financial reasons. It is a widespread practice that has existed for many years in the US. As early as the late 1800s, *The New York Times* published an exposé about private New York hospitals using ambulances to shift poor patients to Bellevue, a public hospital.[25] Over the years, it has become increasingly institutionalized as part of our health care system and yet remains a discomforting fact that garners intermittent and unwanted attention for private hospitals and the larger health care system. More recently, Congress passed the Emergency Medical Treatment and Active Labor Act (EMTALA), a federal anti-dumping legislation, as part of the Consolidated Omnibus Budget Reconciliation Act of 1986 (COBRA) in response to public outrage over hospitals dumping or forcing out uninsured patients. EMTALA mandates hospitals to "stabilize" a patient with an emergency medical condition, regardless of the patient's ability to pay or their citizenship status, and only transfer or discharge that patient to an "appropriate" medical facility.[26] However, it is largely a limited measure that restricts hospitals from transferring a medically indigent[27] patient while they are unstable. Once the patient is stable, the hospital can transfer the patient for any reason, including for purely economic purposes.

Fulfilling the requirements of EMTALA is particularly difficult with respect to undocumented migrants with severe injuries, since "appropriate" long-term care facilities are nearly impossible to find.[28] Some hospitals have resorted to deporting these patients to other countries to avoid these costs.[29] Others have tried to avoid admitting these patients into their emergency room in the first place or discharged them to family members as quickly as possible.

Writing shortly after the passage of EMTALA, Enfield and Sklar state that, "while Americans have been loathe to suggest that the quality of health care one receives should depend on one's ability to pay, we have been unable to define health care as a basic right to which all individuals are entitled."[30] The practice of patient dumping makes visible an unequal and segregated system of care, wherein better health care for the wealthy is bolstered by shifting uncompensated costs (and people) to hospitals that can least afford it. Safety net hospitals bear a deeply unequal burden of these costs. A series of key studies in the 1980s demonstrated the severe impact of this practice on low-income communities and public hospitals across the nation. One study found that among 458 patients transferred from other hospitals to the Highland General Hospital emergency department in Oakland, California, 63% had no insurance, 34% had Medicaid or Medicare, and only 3% had private insurance.[31] Another study of hospital transfers to Cook County Hospital in Chicago found that 87% of these patients were uninsured and 89% were Black or Latino.[32]

Still another study of hospital transfers to the emergency department at Regional Medical Center in Memphis, Tennessee, found 91% were sent for primarily economic reasons, and one out of four were clinically unstable upon arrival.[33] In addition to increased health risks for the patient, this study documents other consequences that accompany patient dumping. First, patients were charged for the ambulance ride from the private hospital to the public hospital and a second emergency department evaluation upon arrival. Relatedly, Enfield and Sklar note the common practice of private hospitals to tell medically indigent patients "how much their medical care will cost, and then to suggest that the patient would be better off at the county hospital because treatment there would be free."[34] This statement is incorrect and misleading. The researchers found that the care provided at the county hospital cost as much as, if not more than, what the transferring private hospital would charge. They write, "Most patients at county hospitals are billed for services rendered. Those that are not must qualify under local and state indigent programs to receive free services. Such programs exclude significant numbers of the medically indigent, such as working people who are underinsured or uninsured."[35] Second, the shifting of costs to public hospitals increases inequality by enriching the budget of private hospitals while destabilizing the financial health of public hospitals. In Memphis, Kellermann and Hackman estimate that more than $1.3 million in uncompensated care was absorbed by the publicly subsidized Regional Medical Center (Med) from local private hospitals transfers during their three-month-long study. They write,

Defenders of "economic transfers" in Shelby County argue that since the Med is the only hospital treating adults in Memphis to receive a direct operating subsidy, it bears sole responsibility for the care of indigent county citizens. This assertion ignores the fact that Shelby County's annual subsidy of $26.8 million covers less than half of the uncompensated care provided by our institution.[36]

During the year of the study (1986), the Med reported a net operating deficit of $7 million. This is in stark contrast to the private hospitals of Shelby County, which reported net revenues in 1986 (following allowances for bad debt and charity care) of $62 million.[37] The authors also note that as "charitable institutions," all but one of these private hospitals were exempt from county taxes.[38] This example shows how different sources of government funding are used to support both public and private health care institutions (albeit at different rates), but private hospitals appear to largely circumvent the expectations accompanying public subsidies. And, in response to those who defend patient dumping as a financial necessity in the face of intense economic pressures facing the health care marketplace, the authors state,

> In many cases, the financial pressures cited as justification for patient dumping are not as great as are commonly thought. For example, had the private hospitals of Memphis kept all of the patients described in our study, their net revenues (following all allowances for bad debt and charity care) would have been decreased by less than 2 percent. Financial considerations should not absolve any institution or individual of their fundamental obligation to render medically necessary emergency treatment.[39]

This case study is an important example of how panic regarding health care expenditure, particularly around indigent care, can conveniently obscure the financial reality of hospitals and provide cover for its unjust institutional practices.

In assessing the larger consequences of patient dumping, Enfield and Sklar argue that the state of American medicine as a two-tiered delivery system is exacerbated through this practice, and it goes against the commonplace aspiration in the US that the quality of medical care should not depend on one's ability to pay.[40] They write, "It became an embarrassment which the federal government addressed when the cut-throat climate of medicine, coupled with significant documentation of the serious consequences of patient dumping in the press and medical literature, began to erode public confidence in the medical profession."[41] Unfortunately, this embarrassment continues despite legislations like EMTALA, and makes worse the inequalities of health care beyond the Second Net, into the Third Net.

The Third Net is a result of patient dumping. While dramatic in its visual representation of injustice, patient dumping is a foreseeable by-product of a market approach to health care that allows the upper tiers to discriminate on the basis of class, race, and immigration status and then shift those they do not want to the informal Third Net. Consequently, while the inverted pyramid of figure I.4 illustrates the clear hierarchy of the US health care system, there is also regular movement across the stratified categories. At the same time, organizations in the Third Net regularly engage the core safety net, and even the private sector, should an opportunity arise. For instance, some volunteer staff of the Third Net may be formally employed by local hospitals and draw on their personal connections to provide patients access to specialty care within the First or Second Net.

If measured by finances and human resources, the Third Net is minuscule in comparison, but its position is critical in absorbing the inherent inequality of the US health care system and thereby softening its impact. It appears that a "dumping ground" of those excluded, as unsightly as it may seem, is an essential part of the overall functioning of the health care system.

Infrastructure of the Third Net, Part I: Public Charge

There is no exact definition of what constitutes "infrastructure." What makes something or someone "essential" to modern state governance could vary, given that it is relational and ecological—meaning, a technology may be viewed as necessary for the governance of a particular context or environment but not another. There is no universal tool, just as there is no universal condition. According to Susan Leigh Star, "it means different things to different groups and it is part of the balance of action, tools, and the built environment."[42] It involves such mundane things as levers, codes of behavior or standards, and bureaucratic forms.

This is an apt description of the Third Net of the health care safety net. The infrastructure of the Third Net comprises an informal cadre of volunteers with a wide range of strategies, resources, and experiences, who provide basic care in ways that reflect the political and social conditions of their region. Studying the mundane mechanisms of infrastructure from different vantage points reveals the patterns and particular processes of how a system operates, providing an opportunity to critically reassess its components and the ways in which it can be restructured.

An infrastructural framework, as outlined by Appel, Anand, and Gupta,[43] allows us to "defamiliarize and rethink" components of health care provision as an essential part of governance. Fundamentally, the study of infrastructure is the study of social relations; more specifically, it is an articulation of power, politics, and its contestations. In our analysis, we focus on the health care providers who serve migrants to understand how the safety net operates—the technological mechanisms, bureaucratic partnerships, and paradoxical politics that both fortify its foundation and signal its disintegration.

Nikhil Anand argues in *Hydraulic City*, "The city and its citizens are made and unmade by the everyday practices around water provisioning—practices that are as much about slaking thirst as they are about making durable forms of belonging in the city."[44] Similarly, the social life of health care infrastructure also tells us how everyday forms of membership or lack thereof are constructed. Here, we are particularly interested in the production of migrants as burdensome outsiders through health care. In his study of Mumbai's water distribution, Anand found that semiotic and material conditions of daily management are unstable and, many times, of multiple and potentially contradictory historical, social, and material relations.[45] Anand writes, "Infrastructures are flaky accretions of sociomaterial processes that are brought into being through relations with human bodies, discourses, and other things (sewage, soil, water, filtration plants). They are processes always in formation and . . . always coming apart."[46] In this way, infrastructure is understood as social processes that are always in the making, purposefully incomplete, and on the verge of falling apart. Again, this aptly characterizes the persistent state of the US health care system and the multiple layers of the fraying safety net. It is a hierarchical process that shifts with the people, politics, and larger social contexts of a particular place. At the same time, there is an order and purpose to this seeming disarray, or patchwork, of parts.

The health care system, including practitioners in the Third Net, plays a critical role in regulating the everyday lives of people in poverty. As social scientists have convincingly articulated, the goal of poverty governance is not to eliminate poverty but rather to manage the poor into docile and industrious subjects.[47] The invaluable condition of health, along with the elevated social status and moral authority attributed to health care providers, allows for extraordinary disciplinary powers. At the same time, there are variations in the use of this power across the tiers of the health care infrastructure. Within the Third Net, health care safety net practitioners function as "street-level bureaucrats," who play a unique role in poverty governance. Rather than a Weberian vision of bureaucracy as a strict system of super- and subordination where street-level bureaucrats execute the state's demands,[48] health care providers in the Third Net are frontline workers who bridge gaps in the health care infrastructure. As chapter 1 illustrates, these street-level bureaucrats leverage their networks and relationships to facilitate access to resources, and in this way, they are influenced by but not entirely beholden to the state's authority.[49] At the same time, their extreme marginality (or near absence) as part of the larger health care infrastructure also serves as a challenge to the system itself. Through their labor, they have the capacity to negotiate a middle ground between the demands of the state from above and needs of the indigent from below, but with their own set of motivations (further details are provided in chapter 2).

For low-income migrants, poverty governance is also reinforced through immigration enforcement—of particular note is public charge.[50] Public charge is an administrative law that allows for the exclusion of migrants through inadmission or deportation, based on a discretionary determination of an individual's potential to become a public burden. As chapter 4 makes clear, public charge is a convenient and powerful tool to control the movement of migrants and discipline their behavior, and it has served as a driving force in the national outcry against the presence of migrants in the US. The US has had in place a "public charge" provision within immigration law, adapted from English poor laws, that allows for the exclusion of those migrants deemed a burden upon the state. The popularity of this administrative law as a bureaucratic tool of exclusion and deportation has ebbed and flowed for over a hundred years. More recently, it has served as an effective tool in justifying the dumping of patients deemed burdensome by the formal safety net to the Third Net.

In the 1990s, the growing visible presence of migrants, particularly those from Latin America, triggered a series of onslaughts to destabilize the migration flow. As part of this politically charged environment, low-income migrants were continuously characterized as burdensome, unwanted dependents on US society by elected officials and conservative media institutions. This was a powerful and effective campaign of dehumanization and criminalization, in part because it followed a familiar message perfected earlier with the myth of the Black "welfare queen" as a poverty governance strategy.[51]

The ideology of public charge is present in many landmark welfare, immigration, and health care legislations. For instance, the federal welfare reform bill (PRWORA—Personal Responsibility and Opportunity for Work Reform Act—PL 104–193), which profoundly diminished the US welfare state, disproportionately targeted migrants. Almost 50% of the initial cuts in this major federal legislation were directed at the limited services available for migrants living in poverty. Then, a month later, the federal immigration legislation (IIRIRA—Illegal Immigration Reform and Immigrant Responsibility Act—PL 104–208) also passed. Both of these federal policies explicitly linked immigration status to eligibility for public benefits by creating new categories of exclusion.[52] The repeated mention of "responsibility" in the title of both policies is noteworthy, as it stresses the goal of regulating and inducing particular behavior defined as "responsible" upon those populations already assumed to be irresponsible.

The passage of the two federal welfare and immigration laws also facilitated the exchange of information regarding individual applicants across different governmental agencies. For instance, PRWORA explicitly prohibits the use of federal funds for Medicaid benefits other than emergency care for specific groups of migrants. Therefore, unless they have a specific, verifiable immigration status, migrants are only allowed coverage for emergency care. States must now verify the immigration status of a foreign-born Medicaid applicant with Immigration and

Customs Enforcement (ICE) if the person applies for a Medicaid benefit that includes federal financial participation.[53]

Further, public charge law and sentiment functions as a foundational apparatus for maintaining "illegality," a juridical status and sociolegal condition that keeps migrants deportable and exploitable.[54] Since 1965, these powerful immigration tools of poverty governance have disproportionately targeted Latinx communities in the US. As Bacong and Menjívar assert, "The immigration system is itself racialized, based on seemingly neutral laws that target Latinas/os, making them synonymous with being undocumented."[55] The immigration status of "undocumented" or "illegal" has become racialized as Latinx, and subsequently led to greater discrimination and criminalization, and contributed to greater stress and poorer health.[56] In fact, the racialization of undocumented legal status is so strong that studies have found a "spillover" effect in which all Latinx, regardless of actual legal status, are negatively impacted. At the same time, given the absence of discussion of undocumented Asians, it comes as a shock to know that one out of every seven Asian migrants is undocumented, making Asians the fastest-growing group of undocumented migrants in the US.[57] Bacong and Menjívar write, "As a result, many illegalized Asians may be deterred from seeking health care and social services for fear of outing their legal status or because they believe that there may be no resources catering to their community."[58]

Currently, the Latinx population is the largest racial/ethnic minority group in the US and a significant portion of this population are migrants (34%).[59] There are also an estimated 11.3 million undocumented migrants in the US, and most are from Mexico and countries in Central America (El Salvador, Guatemala, Nicaragua, and Honduras). In a systematic review of research studies on the health-related effects of punitive immigration policies, Nicholas Vernice and colleagues found that "the U.S. is unquestionably experiencing heightened anti-immigrant sentiment."[60] Their review notes the particular harm of a "new era of public charge" to health equity and concludes that "many punitive immigrant policies have decreased immigrant access to and utilization of basic health care services, while instilling fear, confusion, and anxiety in these communities."[61]

Relatedly, Heide Castañeda and colleagues argue that given the enormous consequences of immigration status on daily life, it is an important social determinant of health.[62] Going beyond serving as a "protective factor" or a "stressor" on individuals, it has a structural effect that is central to health conditions produced and reproduced by larger social and economic inequalities. Key studies, which laid the foundations of this research area, include Nancy Krieger's[63] publications on the "eco-social," Williams's[64] and Takeuchi's[65] research on racism and health disparities, Phelan and Link's[66] theory of "fundamental social causes," and Kawachi and Kennedy's[67] framing of "social determinants of health inequality." These studies have opened our understanding of social inequality as the cause of illness and premature death, and this more expansive understanding of a socially derived cause, coupled with an infrastructural approach, highlights social forces at the structural level as the locus of change in our study. For the Latinx community, race/ethnicity and immigration status remain structurally conflated to the detriment of their health, making clear the racialization of the infrastructure of health care and its disparities. As Edna Viruell-Fuentes et al. noted, "In the popular imagination all Latinos are perceived to be Mexican, all Mexicans are seen as immigrants, and they, in turn, are all cast as undocumented. These conflations mean that anti-immigrant sentiments aimed at undocumented immigrants translate into a hostile environment for entire groups of people, regardless of their immigrant status."[68]

Infrastructure of the Third Net, Part II: Affordable Care Act

The primary purpose of the Affordable Care Act (ACA) was to extend health insurance to the 49 million uninsured people in the US. By 2016, more than 18 million non-elderly adults gained insurance, amounting to a 46% reduction in the number of non-elderly adults without insurance.[69] Beyond these numbers, virtually the entire US population is affected to some extent by its many provisions, including new rules for private insurance and existing public insurance programs that extend patient protections and increase affordability for health care.[70]

For undocumented migrants, however, the ACA doubled down on their exclusion. On the face of it, the ACA should not affect undocumented migrants at all. As noted earlier, undocumented migrants were ineligible for public health insurance coverage prior to the ACA and remained so after the ACA. With the ACA, they are not only ineligible for public health insurance but are also restricted from purchasing private health insurance at full cost in state insurance exchanges. The only health insurance options for undocumented migrants are 1) to voluntarily purchase insurance in the private insurance market outside of state exchanges in states where one exists (and without state subsidies or tax credits to offset these costs), or 2) to get an employer-sponsored plan, when available. Many undocumented migrants find the costs prohibitive since these products are not federally subsidized, and most low-income migrants work in industries where employer-sponsored insurance is not an option. These restrictions result in undocumented migrants remaining uninsured at five times the rate of US-born citizens and less likely to obtain needed care or preventative services.

For the majority of undocumented migrants, health care access is restricted to emergency care and, when available, non-emergency health services at community health centers or safety net hospitals.[71] Even with their limited access to care, however, noncitizen adults and children are less likely than citizens to seek care from an emergency room. In 2010, migrants were nearly half as likely as citizens to visit an emergency room for care.[72] On average, they have lower per capita health care costs than US citizens and legal residents. Although undocumented migrants represent 12% of the non-elderly adult population, they account for only 6% of health spending.[73] Undocumented migrants tend to be younger working adults who are uninsured and avoid using health care as much as possible.

In a health economics study, Brown, Wilson, and Angel found that excluding undocumented male migrants from Mexico from the ACA does not lower medical costs. This is in part because recent migrants are healthier upon arrival than Mexican Americans already residing in the US. Given that the Latinx population uses less health care than non-Latinx Whites, the inclusion of undocumented migrants in an insurance pool could help reduce the premiums of all individuals in an insurance exchange. They write, "Rather than being a burden under the [ACA], including immigrants from Mexico could ease premium costs for citizens, at least in the short term, because relatively healthy people are added to the pool lowering pooled costs."[74] However, public opinion against coverage of undocumented migrants remains as strong as ever. Apparently, access to health care denotes a "public good" that goes beyond an accounting of economic costs. In their deep and increasing marginalization from the formal health care system, undocumented migrants are isolated in the Third Net and thereby "disappeared" from the sphere of the "public."

The Affordable Care Act fundamentally changed the entire health care landscape, but safety net hospitals and clinics have faced greater challenges in comparison to the private sector. And within the safety net sector, the ACA's impact on a hospital or clinic is largely determined by the state in which it resides and whether or not their policymakers decided to expand eligibility for Medicaid. Studies show that safety net hospitals in states that did expand Medicaid now treat more insured and fewer uninsured patients after the ACA, and this change has significantly improved their financial outlook.[75] Despite initial concerns that safety net hospitals would lose many newly insured patients to other private-sector providers, these safety net hospitals were able to not only retain existing patients but also gain newly insured patients, especially for their outpatient care. Efforts to help uninsured patients enroll in coverage, expand primary care capacity, and improve their facilities and systems to attract new patients proved successful for safety net providers in states like California and Arizona.[76] Overall, although they experienced some decline in federal subsidies for indigent care and continue to worry about further funding cuts in the future, the greater numbers of insured patients through the ACA have financially improved these First and Second Net core health care providers.

It is a different story for safety net hospitals in Texas, which did not expand Medicaid. Hospitals like Harris Health in Houston experienced little change in the number of insured patients while dealing with increasing financial challenges. Texas had the highest population of uninsured residents in the country prior to the ACA and remained so after the ACA. Leading up to the Affordable Care Act, Harris Health had optimistically invested significant funds to build its primary care capacity. Using Delivery System Reform Incentive Payment or "DSRIP" waivers, a program funded by Medicaid to support hospitals that serve large numbers of uninsured patients, Harris Health increased its patient volume by opening nine primary care clinics, which subsequently increased demand for specialty services. At the same time, county tax support, which accounts for 47% of its operating revenue, and Medicaid

Disproportionate Share Hospital (DSH) payments, an important federal funding source, decreased in anticipation of Medicaid expansion.

When Medicaid expansion did not happen, Harris Health experienced significant financial losses—$24 million in 2013, $17 million in 2014, and $14 million in 2015—as it tried to adjust to the reality of increased uncompensated care of 12% and decreased DSH payments of 13%, along with the loss of county support totaling $75 million since 2011.[77] By refusing to participate in ACA Medicaid expansion, Texas forced its safety net hospitals to endure continued financial insecurity. Hospitals such as Harris Health must rely on federal funding from alternative sources such as DSRIP waivers and anxiously hope for its periodic renewal, while bracing for expected ACA-related cuts in Medicaid DSH payments. The federal government plans to significantly reduce Medicaid DSH payments in the coming years.[78]

Clearly, the Affordable Care Act has changed the bureaucratic infrastructure of the health care safety net, and individual state decisions to expand Medicaid eligibility created distinct variations in how different regions adapted to these changes. However, what remained consistent was the impetus for patient dumping to the Third Net. States such as Arizona, which expanded Medicaid eligibility, as well as states like Texas, which did not, focused their efforts on increasing the number of insured patients while decreasing the number of those uninsured—albeit under significantly different circumstances.

In our interviews, community outreach workers in the formal First and Second Nets noted greater marginalization of low-income undocumented migrants as a patient population for many safety net hospitals and clinics as they focused their attention on those who are eligible for coverage under the ACA. Other studies report similar effects. Marrow and Joseph[79] describe heightened conditions of uncertainty in which health and immigration policy concerns overlap, and Van Natta[80] found that even for safety net hospitals and clinics within supportive local communities with strong policies and institutional commitments to serve vulnerable patients, low-income and undocumented migrants were unable to fully access care. They report unnecessary levels of morbidity and mortality for this population as a result of structural barriers and federal legislation and, in some cases, "patients returned to their country of origin to die."[81]

Health Care Safety Net in Phoenix, Arizona

In January 2012, Arizona's Republican Governor Jan Brewer became the figurehead for conservative opposition to President Obama, when she wagged her finger at him during an intense conversation on the tarmac in Mesa, Arizona.[82] Just 18 months later, however, Governor Brewer expended much political capital within her party to lobby for support among Republican state legislators for Medicaid expansion under the Affordable Care Act, even after Arizona was one of the plaintiffs in the unsuccessful Supreme Court challenge to the ACA.[83] Perhaps the most outspoken Republican governor in favor of expanding Medicaid, Brewer was one of only 11 Republican governors in the US to decide to take up this provision of the ACA.[84] As a result, upwards of 300,000 uninsured Arizonans became eligible for health coverage under the Arizona Health Care Cost Containment System (AHCCCS), Arizona's Medicaid program.[85] Following its initial passing, Brewer's Medicaid expansion plan faced a number of legal challenges from Republican lawmakers in the state that opposed this expansion.[86]

Although the state expanded Medicaid, Arizona did not adopt the second major provision of the ACA—the creation of a state-run marketplace. In April 2015, Republican Governor Doug Ducey, who succeeded Brewer for governor, cited his opposition to "Obamacare" when he signed a bill into law that banned Arizona from creating a state-run health marketplace.[87] As a result, Arizonans must rely on the federal Health Insurance Marketplace to purchase health coverage. This law also attempted to take away health insurance subsidies from Arizonans who purchased health coverage from the federal marketplace, but the Supreme Court declared this part of the law unconstitutional when it issued a ruling upholding subsidies regardless of whether a state operates its own health marketplace or not.[88]

By the end of 2016, the uninsurance rate in Arizona had fallen by almost 40%, with roughly an additional 140,000 people accessing health insurance through the marketplace.[89] In each the fiscal years of 2014 and 2015, Medicaid enrollment also increased by roughly 20%,[90] and by May 2017, Medicaid enrollment was at half a million more enrolled and insured Arizonans than pre-ACA (1.2 million and 1.7 million respectively).[91] As of August 2022, this number has grown to over 2.4 million people.[92] Overall, the story of the ACA in Arizona is echoed around the country (especially in states that expanded Medicaid): the ACA has dramatically increased access to health insurance coverage for the poorest Arizonans who were unable to afford insurance or care and/ or were previously ineligible for Medicaid. Rates of uninsurance in the state have fluctuated since the dramatic dip that accompanied the ACA's implementation in 2014.[93] As premium costs have steadily and swiftly increased, uninsurance rates have also increased as individuals opted to pay the tax penalty for not being insured rather than paying the cost of the premiums. In fact, from 2016 to 2017, the premiums for a benchmark plan in Phoenix more than doubled from $207 to $507 (although this difference was largely covered by tax credits for those who were eligible for them).[94]

The state has several large hospitals and medical centers that provide care to Arizonans, especially in the two largest counties—Maricopa County, with Phoenix as the largest metro area, and Pima County, with Tucson as the second-largest city in the state. The fifth-largest city in the US, behind Houston, Phoenix sprawls across an over-500-square mile area that is larger than Los Angeles or Chicago. Additionally, the greater Phoenix metro area comprises more than 20 smaller cities and towns, and it is often hard to distinguish the boundaries between the incorporated area of the city and these other cities and towns, which include considerable cities in their own right like Tempe and Mesa. Almost 20% of Phoenix residents are foreign-born, and over half of the migrants living in Phoenix are from Mexico.[95] Phoenix is home to a number of large medical systems and hospitals, FQHCs, public and community health organizations, and nonprofit and free clinics. These include Banner University Medical Center, which is affiliated with the University of Arizona College of Medicine, which is the largest hospital in the state and a nonprofit research and teaching hospital. St. Joseph's Hospital is a Catholic nonprofit hospital in Phoenix with a Level I trauma center and a specialty in neurology.

Although these two large hospitals provide some safety net care to indigent patients, the main safety net hospital system in Maricopa County is called Valleywise Health (formerly Maricopa Medical Center), a consortium of hospitals and health centers that include a Level I trauma center, a Level III neonatal intensive care unit (NICU), and the state's only burn unit. Maricopa County originally oversaw Maricopa Medical Center, but in 2003, voters approved the creation of the Maricopa County Special Health Care District, which assumed oversight of the hospital system in 2005. The district's five directors are elected officials who maintain oversight of the state's only public health care system. They have the power, authority, and responsibility to evaluate "(1) revenue sources and how they are used; (2) fiscal condition and changes needed to ensure financial stability; (3) executive management salaries and how they compare nationally; (4) contract personnel and costs; (5) the amount of medical services provided to indigent individuals and policies governing those services; and (6) the amount of uncompensated care provided."[96] At its creation, voters also authorized the district's board with the power to levy taxes to maintain fiscal viability for the health system, and the board implemented a second property tax in 2006 that raised about $40 million for the health system. The board represents a unique management and public oversight arrangement for the county's safety net health care system, and the shift to district board supervision has moved the hospital system from the red to the black with a much more auspicious fiscal future.

Health Care Safety Net in Houston, Texas

Located in Harris County, Houston is the fourth-largest city in the country, with approximately 2.2 million residents. From 1970 to 2000, the population of Harris County doubled, largely due to immigration. As a result, Houston is the most ethnically and culturally diverse area in the nation;[97] 25% percent of Harris County residents are foreign-born, 70% of whom are from Latin America and another 21% from Asia. Harris County is home to an array of primary, secondary, and tertiary health care resources. In fact, the Houston metropolitan region is home to the largest medical center in the world, the Texas Medical Center, with some of the nation's best hospitals and physicians. An internationally recognized health care facility, the Medical Center includes 21 hospitals and receives over 7 million visits a year.[98] Paradoxically, roughly one-third of Harris County residents rely on safety net providers, including emergency rooms, for their health care needs. These safety net providers that work with specific underserved communities include 10 FQHCs, public health and community health organizations, and medical school partners (Baylor College of Medicine, UT Medical School at Houston, and UT Houston Health Science Center), and a large network of health care providers under the umbrella of the Harris Health System, a large public health care system in Harris County.

In attempts to mitigate some of the health needs of the uninsured, the Harris Health System provides the vast majority of the safety net health care provision in the county, offering primary, specialty, and acute care to uninsured and low-income patients. Harris Health is not only the largest source of health care for low-income and uninsured patients, it is also one of the largest public hospital systems in the country. In addition to operating the three main public hospitals (Ben Taub, Lyndon B. Johnson, and Quentin Mease) in Harris County, Harris Health manages 19 community health centers and numerous other clinics and programs situated across the region. In 2016, 91.9% of patients seen at Harris Health were either uninsured (62.4%) or covered by Medicaid and CHIP (20.4%) or Medicare (9.5%), and 88.8% of these patients identified as an ethnic/racial minority.[99] In the past, Harris Health quietly included undocumented migrants as part of its patient population but, during the initial implementation stage of the ACA, a significant amount of energy and resources were concentrated on the enrollment of eligible patients into the ACA. As a result, particular concerns of undocumented migrants fell further from its central mission and a number of community organizations tried to fill the unmet health care needs of those who cannot access formal medical institutions.

Since Texas opposed the implementation of the two most prominent components of the federal Affordable Care Act (the expansion of Medicaid and the creation of a state-level Health Insurance Marketplace), the federal Department of Health and Human Services (DHHS) operates a federally facilitated health insurance marketplace for Texans. Furthermore, as a result of this decision, Texas was not eligible for federal funds that would have covered 100% of the cost of Medicaid expansion for the first three years and approximately 90% in subsequent years. These decisions left uninsured 1.5 million non-disabled adults below 138% of the federal poverty level who would have been eligible for health coverage under Medicaid expansion.

By February 2016, over 1.2 million Texans had enrolled in health insurance through the federal ACA marketplace. Consequently, the uninsured rate of 27% in 2013 declined to 17.3% in 2020. Texas has twice the national average of uninsured people, at 17.3%, which is 3 percentage points more than Oklahoma, the state with the next-highest uninsurance rate.[100] And, within Texas, the 29th Congressional District has the highest uninsurance rate in the country, at 31%. The 29th Congressional District encompasses the eastern portion of the Greater Houston area and is located in Harris County.

Methods

We began our study at a critical moment. The Affordable Care Act came into full effect in 2014 as we entered our fieldwork. Enrollments opened for newly mandated Health Insurance Marketplaces (also called exchanges), and all citizens who met certain income thresholds were required to purchase some form of coverage. Health insurance is a critical determinant in accessing health care and improving health equity, and millions of people benefited from the ACA as the number of uninsured nonelderly Americans fell from over 48 million in 2010 to 28 million in 2016.[101] However, these benefits were unevenly distributed. Ye and Rodriguez's study of health insurance coverage found that migrants—particularly those with low English proficiency, which could indicate relatively recent migration to the US and/or workforce participation in low-income, low-status, segregated labor—experienced the least benefits from the ACA.[102] Structural vulnerabilities existing prior to the ACA were evident after the ACA.

Our study supports and extends this finding. An infrastructural focus on the everyday practice of health care providers in the Third Net reveals how the conditions of explicit exclusion—of both restrictive health care policy and draconian immigration enforcement—within the formal safety net are built against low-income migrants. It is worth repeating that the explicit exclusion of undocumented migrants from the ACA allowed for its passage. In this way, the exclusion of undocumented migrants was directly tied to the expansion of Medicaid to millions of low-income citizens. At the same time, the Third Net is pivotal to the system overall, serving to buttress the formal First and Second

Nets. As the "dumping ground" for the health care system, the Third Net has been critical in masking the unseemly conditions of its overall systemic infrastructure. As our study will show, low-income migrants did not simply fall through the cracks of a "broken" health care system. Rather, the health care infrastructure was purposely created to externalize migrant health care to the Third Net.

It is within this precarious health care safety net, after decades of dwindling public health support, welfare retrenchment, and neoliberal economic policies, that we faced the COVID-19 pandemic. While there is much to unpack (for years to come) in understanding the many impacts of this global health crisis, the most obvious observation is that we were ill-prepared. And perhaps the second obvious point is that those most vulnerable within unequal systems have borne and will bear the brunt of the pandemic. From an infrastructural analysis, it is evident that the lack of preparation and exacerbation of vulnerabilities is structurally conditioned and predictable. As David Harvey notes,

> Public authorities and health care systems were almost everywhere caught short-handed. Forty years of neoliberalism across North and South America and Europe had left the public totally exposed and ill-prepared to face a public health crisis of this sort, even though previous scares of SARS and Ebola provided abundant warnings as well as cogent lessons as to what would be needed to be done.[103]

The COVID-19 pandemic also revealed the key role of low-income, undocumented migrants, as those with the least amount of protection against the virus, in upholding social systems deemed "essential." This is a governmental national security designation dating from the Cold War; essential workers are those working in particular industrial and service sectors deemed critical. There are an estimated 50 to 60 million people in the US who hold jobs categorized as essential to "continued infrastructure viability."[104] Within recent COVID-19 conditions, this has meant that those already made vulnerable by social inequality are forced to endure greater risk of exposure so that those with greater privilege will not. One study found that residents of low-income, non-white counties were nearly eight times more likely to be infected with COVID-19 than residents of low-income, predominantly white counties.[105]

Our study outlines the infrastructure of the health care safety net leading up to COVID-19 and the pivotal role of the Third Net in upholding the overall social safety net. In this regard, the heightened role of low-income undocumented migrants as crucial, or "essential," workers foundational for the operation of larger society is not surprising. What is also not surprising is the continued hostility in immigration enforcement and restrictive access to health care for these same essential workers. Regardless of how illogical and ill-prepared the US may be in meeting the challenges of a systemic crisis, the current infrastructure with all its inequalities functions to benefit powerful entities.

From the vantage point of the Third Net, the US health system, organized in a rigid hierarchy dictated by financing sources, appears to require a precarious Third Net at the bottom. While it is generally agreed that Latinx, African American, Pacific Islander, and Indigenous communities have been disproportionately ravaged, and poverty-driven health impairments and "essential" employment have made some people more vulnerable, critical race scholars have had to repeatedly explain that the disproportionate rates of COVID-19 are *not* a result of innate racial differences or "race," but rather that the problem is "racism." In a recent issue of *Science* (September 11, 2020), Michael Yudell, Dorothy Roberts, and colleagues wrote, "Although genetic risk factors may contribute to severity of COVID-19, race is a poor proxy to understand the population distribution of such risk factors. Compelling evidence shows that racism, not race, is the most relevant risk factor."[106] In addition, in 2020, the Centers for Disease Control identified racism as a "serious public health threat,"[107] defining racism as "a system—consisting of structures, policies, practices, and norms—that assigns value and determines opportunity based on the way people look or the color of their skin." The infrastructure of the health care safety net is clearly a key research site to understand how such systems of inequality continue to function.

This study began with the intent to assess the effects of the ACA for undocumented migrants in four states along the southern US border between 2014 and 2016. The initial rollout of the Affordable Care Act (ACA) was tumultuous. The seemingly continuously changing rules associated with this major federal policy, in conjunction with sharp variations in individual states' responses, created significant challenges for health care providers. Consequently, the multiple methods for this study were designed to capture the unpredictability of this process and allow for potentially unforeseen changes.

As our study progressed, our interests broadened beyond the ACA, as we began to see the outlines of an infrastructure within a messy, informal landscape of the safety net system. At the same time, we saw the need for multiple methods—combining semi-structured interviews with key respondents across multiple states and regions with in-depth ethnographies at specific Third Net organizations in two different states—to provide a rich description of the infrastructure from the vantage point of those within it.

We first identified safety net hospitals and clinics and migrant health advocates in four metropolitan areas—Houston, Texas; Albuquerque, New Mexico; Phoenix Arizona; and San Diego, California—that serve large numbers of migrant patients. We focused on these US-Mexico border states, which have each garnered considerable public attention for their politics and policies surrounding immigration and migrants. We visited each site, conducting in-person interviews with key respondents.[108]

The selection of key respondents relied on a combination of sampling procedures. Careful literature, media, and internet searches on migrant health care access, along with conversations with knowledgeable policy researchers, helped identify the initial pool of potential interviewees. Introducing our study as an assessment of institutions' responses to changes in the safety net since the passing of the ACA, we contacted key individuals—administrators, health care providers, and community health advocates—in hospitals, clinics, and community organizations via telephone and email and employed a snowball sampling technique for the recruitment of additional participants. In this process, we expanded our interviews to Tucson, Arizona, as its significance became evident in our understanding of the Third Net in Arizona and, at the same, we decided to pull San Diego so that we may devote greater attention to our Arizona and Texas research sites. In the first year of the study, we recruited and conducted a total of 42 face-to-face in-depth interviews with health care providers and migrant advocacy organizations.

A year later, we conducted a second set of interviews. We reinterviewed the initial respondents to gauge any changes over the year as well as interviewed additional hospital personnel and migrant community advocates in Phoenix, Tucson, and Houston. In all, we conducted a total of 112 interviews from 2014 to 2016. The interviews centered topically on the health care safety net, state and local politics, private hospital systems, and the ACA, and they ranged from in-depth, structured interviews lasting two hours or more to relatively brief, semi-structured interviews lasting 30 minutes. Most interviews were conducted in small groups of two to three respondents.

After these interview rounds, we decided to split up and initiate in-depth, year-long ethnographies of two social justice organizations to detail the infrastructural workings of the Third Net. Having acquainted ourselves with the various Third Net organizations in our initial sample, we chose to focus our attention on the CommUnity Clinic of Phoenix (CommUnity Clinic or CCP)[109] in Arizona and Justicia y Paz (Justicia) in Houston, from 2015 to 2016. Each provided a compelling yet distinct example of a migrant health clinic in two states that have large concentrations of migrants and an outsized influence on hostile federal immigration policy. In our fieldwork, we participated in a range of organizational activities, including medical intakes, (in)formal meetings, recreational outings, volunteer orientations, training workshops, and fundraising events. During these activities, we observed volunteer-migrant interactions, points of contention among volunteers, and migrants' medical experiences. After developing rapport, we used a snowball sampling approach to recruit potential interviewees.

In our ethnographies with the two organizations, we conducted 52 in-depth, semi-structured interviews with volunteers who worked in multiple capacities (e.g., health practitioners, interpreters, social workers, etc.). The multi-sited nature of this research was analytically valuable because it allowed us to compare and contrast.[110] We then conducted a thematic analysis[111] of the ethnographic and interview data using NVivo and ATLAS.ti, and by hand. We created thematic reports that noted patterns derived inductively from the analysis and we met repeatedly to discuss our initial results, in an effort to collectively analyze the major themes. Each co-author took responsibility for specific themes and continued to revise and develop these thematic reports into book chapters.

Book Outline

The goal of this book is to articulate the existence of a Third Net and its role as a "dumping ground" undergirding the formal health care system.

While scholarship abounds in describing particular facets of migrant health care, and the larger health care safety net system, we extend this literature by outlining the infrastructure in which these organizations reside. We argue that the Third Net is a critical vantage point from which to understand the purposive disarray of care that is built upon the explicit exclusion of low-income migrants.

Toward this goal, we begin in chapter 1 by analyzing the various Third Net organizations included in this study. Rather than an exhaustive list of health care clinics in the Third Net, our objective is to outline how these organizations can differ from each other. We focus on the multiple philosophies of care and their implications for not only the health services that each provides but the ways in which they are provided. Highlighting the work of five different Third Net organizations in three different counties in Arizona and Texas, this chapter analyzes how the different organizational models affect particular volunteers' negotiation for access to care for their patients and the migrant-provider relationships within them.

Then, chapter 2 delves deeper into one of these organizations, Justicia y Paz. Drawing on interviews and ethnographic observations with volunteers and migrants, health practitioners, and local medical administrators, we argue that Third Net spaces like Justicia survive because they have entire infrastructures of their own. The aim of this chapter is to illustrate the surprisingly extensive infrastructures of support that keep the organization running and growing. In their arduous work of keeping migrants alive, Justicia simultaneously subsidizes ever-shrinking US welfare programs connected to health care, housing, and nutrition assistance. The migrants' stories and experiences and volunteers' insights show how the existence of the Third Net can be read as a critique of the formal US health care system. Our case study of Justicia shows us that we would not need a Third Net if private and safety net hospitals sufficiently addressed existing health disparities.

Chapter 3 continues our in-depth ethnographic inquiry by focusing on CommUnity Clinic of Phoenix. CommUnity shares a social justice philosophy of care similar to that of Justicia, but its free clinic organizational model challenges charity approaches to migrant health care. Its activist history and vision directly critique the systemic failures of the current immigration and health systems as well as other models of free health care based on charity. This chapter outlines the political mission of CommUnity as it negotiates persistent structural constraints in its goal to provide a unique "collage of care." It provides an important example of an alternative, truly non-profit model of care in the midst of an intensely hostile anti-immigrant environment.

Then, in chapter 4, we shift our attention back to Texas with a case study of Houston Health Action (HHA), a distinctive, mutual support–based organization within the Third Net that extends and challenges our understanding of health, care, and migrants. It is a community-based, non-hierarchical group run by and for low-income undocumented migrants with spinal cord injuries. Through a series of interviews with group members and analysis of their website and other related documents pertaining to the group, this chapter analyzes the continued significance of "public charge" as an administrative law and political ideology in the everyday lives of migrants today. We bring together disability and migration studies to understand how public charge functions to justify the exclusion of migrants from the formal health system, funneling them into the informal Third Net.

Finally, the conclusion takes stock of what we have learned about the Third Net and outlines their vision of an alternative health care infrastructure that reimagines what care is and could be. We reiterate the fact that the existence of the Third Net is evidence of the failures of the formal US health care system. At the same time, the Third Net is not accidental or unintentional—it serves a necessary purpose in allowing the US health care system to function as it does. It is also in this site of failure that we see new, albeit imperfect, possibilities.

1

Philosophies of Care

The Third Net is neither homogeneous nor uniform. Though Third Net clinics and organizations share the overall aim of free health care provision for uninsured and often undocumented migrants in the US, they take myriad approaches to this general mission. Various "philosophies of care" examined in this chapter demonstrate these distinct, yet overlapping, approaches. These philosophies of care, which range from traditional charity care to social justice to mutual aid, are evidenced most clearly in the health care services that Third Net organizations provide as well as the ways they communicate their mission and argue for the importance of their work to different stakeholders. This chapter unpacks these various philosophies of care and their implications not only for the health care services of each organization and the way they are provided, but also for framing the work of the Third Net, negotiating health care for patients, shaping patient-provider relationships, and accounting for the role of race in these organizations. Taken together, philosophies of care and their consequences for the work of Third Net organizations demonstrate the infrastructural logics and the potential within the Third Net to envision different configurations of care that address the inequities and injustices of migrant health care and the larger health system in the US.

Specifically, this chapter analyzes the philosophies of care of five different Third Net organizations working across three counties in Arizona and Texas (see table 1.1). Across states and localities, these five organizations provide a representation of the various types of Third Net organizations with varying—yet sometimes overlapping—missions, visions, and approaches to health care.

They all face serious constraints because of the limitations posed, on the one hand, by migrants' ineligibility for health care in the mainstream system and, on the other hand, by the real resource challenges of free health care provision within a larger expensive, privatized health care

TABLE 1.1. Fieldsite organizations (pseudonyms and locations)

Organization (pseudonym)	Centro de Salud	Grace in Action	CommUnity Clinic of Phoenix	Justicia y Paz	Houston Health Action
Informal names and acronyms	Centro	Grace	CommUnity or CCP	Justicia	Health Action or HHA
Locality	Tucson, AZ	Phoenix, AZ	Phoenix, AZ	Houston, TX	Houston, TX

system. As a result, these Third Net organizations are forced to cobble together an infrastructure of preventative, primary, holistic, and specialist care from the expertise and experience of their volunteer health providers and the capabilities of donated (and often outdated) medical equipment. With few to no paid staff, these organizations rely on volunteer health providers, doctors, nurses, dentists, physical therapists, curanderas (spiritual healers), and (aspiring) medical students, to use their knowledge and skills to provide care for thousands of uninsured patients across Arizona and Texas. Beyond the limited services they can provide in house, these organizations heavily rely on their volunteer health providers' social and professional networks of colleagues and like-minded health providers to negotiate through formal and informal channels for more specialized ad hoc, pro bono, and discounted care within the mainstream health system, including screenings and surgeries that these organizations cannot provide on their own. At the same time, hospitals, health care providers, and social service agencies refer a steady stream of patients to these organizations, as they are the only option for health care provision for uninsured, undocumented migrants.

Our cases have similar, yet varied, approaches to the provision of care and thus somewhat different roles and relationships of negotiating access to care and providing medical services to their patients. These differing approaches form a spectrum that demonstrates the multiplicity of missions and frameworks for providing health care in the Third Net. These philosophies of care include traditional charity care, social justice, and mutual aid. (See table 1.2 for a full breakdown of the differences among these organizational philosophies of care, which will be discussed further in this chapter.) Within these overall philosophies, organizations in traditional charity care and social justice also are divided on whether they take a more clinical approach or whether they are modeled more on principles of charity. Some of these organizations are explicitly religiously based and motivated, while others are secular in nature, although they also draw volunteers from various faith traditions. This chapter analyzes the similarities and differences of these various philosophies of care and organizational models and

TABLE 1.2. Philosophies of care in the Third Net

Third Net Philosophies of Care	"Traditional" Charity Care		Social Justice		Mutual Aid
Organizational Model	Free clinic (Centro de Salud)	Charity (Grace in Action)	Free clinic (CommUnity Clinic of Phoenix)	Charity (Justicia y Paz)	Mutual support (Houston Health Action)
Funding Structures	Primarily foundation and government grant funding; some individual donations	Primarily foundation and government grant funding; some individual donations	Primarily individual donations; sometimes limited grant funding	Primarily individual donations; sometimes limited grant funding	Individual donations; member contributions of material goods and skill-sharing
Negotiating Health Care for Patients	Selective referrals into the mainstream system; negotiating discounted and lower-cost care	Formalized partnerships with mainstream health care organizations for referrals	Informal, ad hoc negotiation of care; crowdsourcing more expensive procedures like surgery	Negotiation of care through formal (Harris Gold Card) and informal channels	Ad hoc fundraising and sourcing medical equipment; mutual sharing of health knowledge among members
Framing the Mission	Replicating mainstream clinic model	Replicating traditional charity structure	Envisioning a different model of free health care based on migrant rights and health justice	Envisioning a reality in which migrants' health, material, and spiritual needs are met	Community solidarity and self-determination
Patient-Provider Relationships	Established patient-provider hierarchies that largely replicate mainstream care; volunteer providers motivated by altruism	Established migrant-volunteer hierarchies that mirror traditional charity structure	Intentional work to destabilize patient-provider relationships; migrants as "neighbors" within the same community	Work to challenge migrant-volunteer hierarchies through opening volunteer roles to migrants	Essentially no hierarchy within the organization; all members are also migrants and working to secure each other's health and autonomy

how these impact the services, work, and relationships of Third Net organizations, in particular volunteers' negotiation for access to care for their patients and the migrant-provider relationships within the organizations.

In this chapter and the rest of the book, we examine the work of Third Net organizations largely through the standpoint of the volunteers—including their framing of the organizational vision, their health care provision, and their relationships with patients—in order to understand the different and far-reaching consequences of the various philosophies of care within the Third Net. We engage in an infrastructural analysis of the social relationships in and among migrant health organizations. One of the centrally defining aspects of the Third Net is the way that volunteers must negotiate health care access and provision for patients. In the absence of health insurance coverage and access to affordable health care, community organizations, volunteer health workers, and other individuals rely on their networks and relationships across multiple tiers of the health system to facilitate access to care for uninsured, undocumented migrants. Some scholars have referred to these kinds of relationships as "brokerage," or as a process through which specific actors bridge gaps in social structure by leveraging their networks and relationships to facilitate access to resources.[1] These volunteers can also be understood as "street-level bureaucrats," frontline workers who connect people to social services, knowledge, and robust social networks integral for attaining health care as well as other important social and legal resources.[2] We consider "brokerage" as a shorthand for the relationships that emerge and develop as volunteers and organizations negotiate care for migrant patients or as migrants negotiate care for themselves and others. Our analysis demonstrates that in many ways not addressed by the literature thus far, different forms and relationships of brokerage are the praxis that emerges from an organization's overall philosophy of care. In other words, how these organizations provide and negotiate care for patients is the practice or the work in action of their larger theoretical philosophies of care, and it is in this action that these organizations seek to effect broader social change. For many organizations in our research, these relationships are the means through which they envision and work toward more equitable and just immigration and health systems in the US.

Through analyzing the ways different types of Third Net organizations facilitate health care provision for their patients, we find that, in addition to providing free care within their organizations, volunteers (especially volunteer medical professionals) negotiate ad hoc access to care in the mainstream health system. Beyond the formal and informal relationships between the Third Net and the mainstream health system,[3] some organizations in the Third Net demonstrate radically different discourses and practices of negotiating care for migrant patients.[4] This shift in discourse and practice has the potential to destabilize the power hierarchies of more traditional patient-provider relationships. Our analysis demonstrates ways in which different philosophies of care give rise to different social relationships in the Third Net, which serve not only to facilitate access to the formal health care system but also to establish new health care models more conducive to equitable distributions of power. Negotiating and providing care is not solely about facilitating access to an inequitable medical system for those who have been systematically excluded; it can also involve envisioning and creating more just configurations of care and more equitable migrant-provider relationships.

"Traditional" Approaches to Migrant Health Care in the Third Net

The first philosophy of care is a "traditional" approach to migrant health, which includes the organizational models of a free clinic and a charity. Free clinics and charities with this approach to care are often more publicly visible and generally well known than other organizations of the Third Net. As such, they are often, though not always, more established, larger, and better resourced and connected than other organizations within the Third Net. These organizations may be the recipients of government and large foundation funding and focus their work almost exclusively on the immediate health care and service provision for uninsured (or underinsured) patients. Often this service provision includes patient screenings, primary care, low-cost or free prescription medicines, and health education.

Historically, free medical clinics provided health care services at no cost to their patients, who are uninsured or underinsured and/or otherwise marginalized by the mainstream health system. The existence

of free clinics in the US has radical roots in the New Left social movements and radical health activism of the 1960s and '70s. Many scholars and health movement activists point to the creation of the Haight
Ashbury Free Clinic in 1967 and the Berkeley Free Clinic in 1969 as
sparking the Free Clinic Movement in the US.[5] These early free clinics primarily provided treatment and health care for people who used
drugs and people who distrusted the medical establishment for a variety of reasons. Free clinics and health activism also featured centrally
in the work of radical Civil Rights movement organizations, including
the Black Panthers and the Young Lords as well as the radical feminist
movement.[6] During the '60s and '70s, free medical clinics proliferated
across the US, working to provide care to groups who experienced
medical racism, sexism, and other forms of discrimination in the
mainstream health system. In many ways, these early free clinics (and
some free clinics still today) operated as "outlaw force[s] in medicine."[7]

Once shunned by the American Medical Association (AMA) for
being too radical, free clinics became more mainstream in the 1990s
and received millions of dollars in funding from the AMA and the
Robert Wood Johnson Foundation. This injection of funding led to the
creation of many free clinics around the US, new clinics that often did
not share the radical vision of the early free clinics. In 1996, Congress
passed HIPAA legislation that extended medical malpractice protection
for volunteer professionals working at free clinics, granting additional
legitimacy to and removing some barriers for free clinics. In 2001, the
umbrella organization of the National Association of Free and Charitable Clinics (NAFCC) emerged to represent the over 1,200 free clinics across the US. In 2020, the operating budget for the NAFCC was
over $1.6 million. The NAFCC has received criticism for whitewashing
the radical history and development of the Free Clinic Movement in
order to legitimize its position as representative of free clinics across the
country.[8] The NAFCC has also faced criticism for bureaucratizing and
mainstreaming what was once a radical movement.

With the passage of the Affordable Care Act, many of the former
patients of these free clinics were able to access health insurance. However, free clinics still provide care to millions of people who remain
uninsured and who are undocumented, homeless, unable to afford the
out-of-pocket costs for medical services, and/or living in states that

did not expand Medicaid coverage under the ACA. The majority of the organizations in the Third Net could be considered free clinics or are larger charity organizations that also offer health care as part of their services. However, free clinics have been criticized as a model that is unsustainable within the wider structure and ideology of the mainstream US health care system.[9] Other critics argue that these clinics can reproduce medical hierarchies and even legitimate the current organization of for-profit health care provision in the US.[10] They have also faced pushback for creating a parallel health care system that provides much more limited and inadequate medical services of lower quality than the mainstream system.[11]

In what follows, we introduce the case of Centro de Salud, a free clinic providing health care services, health education, and selective referrals to specialist care for uninsured, undocumented migrants in southern Arizona. As a free clinic, Centro traces its roots to the more recent, mainstream free clinic network that works to model itself as much as possible as a traditional medical clinic, with a few important variations.

Centro de Salud: "Different in All the Right Ways"

Started in 2003 in Tucson, Centro de Salud has provided care to hundreds of low-income, uninsured patients, the vast majority of whom identify as Latinx and many of whom are undocumented migrants who cannot access health care otherwise. The clinic's mission is to "provide quality integrative health services and education at no cost to uninsured and underserved people in a supportive atmosphere." Volunteers at Centro describe their patients as "the most vulnerable members of our community." The majority of the clinic's patients are living with chronic medical conditions like uncontrolled diabetes, high blood pressure, and high cholesterol—all health conditions that are treatable and manageable, but that have often gone without a diagnosis for years. One of the retired doctors who volunteers at the clinic put it this way: "These poor people have absolutely nothing else in the world in the way of health care so we assist them with general maintenance care and as best we can with preventative care. They have literally nothing else for health care."

In order to care for these patients, Centro relies on a cadre of around one hundred volunteers, including retired health professionals, current health workers, medical students at local universities and community colleges, and aspiring medical students who want to work in the health profession in some capacity. In discussing their motivations for volunteering at the clinic, the main themes that emerged were altruistic in nature. One volunteer put it this way: "people come here to help people, and I think that kind of says everything about the people who volunteer here." Additionally, for the retired health professionals, many of whom spend the winters in Tucson as "snowbirds" and then leave for the harsh summers, volunteering at the clinic allows them to continue to practice medicine but in a lower-stress environment; they describe using their skills and expertise to give back and to find purpose in helping patients manage chronic health conditions and health crises. These retired health workers, as well as the current health providers who volunteer at the clinic, often observe firsthand and understand the horror stories of migrants without insurance trying to access care in the mainstream health system. For current and aspiring medical students, volunteering at Centro is often their first real exposure to the clinical setting and the health care system. In addition to patient care, the clinic takes seriously the role it plays in the professional development of future health professionals, working to shape their perspective on their future careers through their work with the clinic's patients.

In many ways, Centro is modeled as a free clinic that mirrors the infrastructure and services of a mainstream clinic, yet it is also shaped by the resource constraints of a clinic working outside of the mainstream system. The clinic started from humble beginnings with little resources and few volunteers, operating outside of regular office hours from a social services building in South Tucson. On clinic days, volunteers arrived to transform the office into a clinic space after social workers left for the day. Out of a large storage closet, volunteers rolled blood pressure machines and carts full of boxes of files into the office lobby to set up for the evening's clinic. Rooms that were used as meeting rooms and offices during the daytime hours quickly transformed into makeshift exam rooms for medical appointments. Students from the local university, some dressed in scrubs, set up a desk for patient check-in and arranged chairs in the front office to form a waiting room for the coming patients, as retired doctors with worn white coats reviewed the files of patients that they were seeing that evening. In the cramped lobby of the office, one volunteer held nutrition education sessions as mothers wrangled and shushed their squirming children while waiting for their appointments.

Centro is not "mobile" in the usual sense of other Third Net organizations housed in a bus or RV that moves from location to location, but, especially in its early days, it was marked by a makeshift mobility and liminality that define so many Third Net organizations. Lacking their own designated offices or clinic spaces, these organizations rely on other spaces for their operations, such as a social services office, a church, or a kitchen in a migrant workers' center. Their internal infrastructure is minimal and nimble. Over the past decades, Centro has grown from the makeshift "mobile" clinic in the social service office in South Tucson to its own designated clinic space. In doing so, it has increased its operating budget by continuing to fundraise individual donations along with being awarded a number of larger grants from foundations and the government. Clinic publicity and volunteer recruitment materials describe a "continuum of care" that combines on-site primary, preventative, specialist, and holistic health care services. Clinic volunteers work to stabilize patients who often have uncontrolled medical situations such as high blood sugar and/or high blood pressure, and then rely on volunteer nutritionists and health educators to help people change their lifestyle and manage their health conditions. Beyond primary care, the services at the clinic include dermatology, ophthalmology, women's health and gynecology, acupuncture, and massage.

Although the organization models itself on a clinic structure, in strategic and important ways the clinic works to address what its volunteers see as some of the barriers or shortcomings of mainstream health clinics. One of the volunteers described their experience with a patient and the work of the clinic: "Recently, a patient told me that Centro is *different in all the right ways*—our volunteers provide stellar patient care in an inviting environment. . . . Knowing that we create a safe and happy space for those who need it most is what Centro is all about" (emphasis added). In other words, the clinic is "different in all the right ways" in the individualized care, welcoming environment, and patient-provider interactions that are intentionally distinct from that in the mainstream health system. In discussing patient-provider interactions, one volunteer noted that "everybody cares about the people that they are helping. All the providers take their time. They're not rushing, and they listen to their patients." Another volunteer described the reluctance of his parents, who were Mexican migrants, to go to a physician as personally motivating for his work at the clinic, where he saw the organization working to "change people's perspective on seeing a physician. My family—being Mexican—they hate going to the physician because they don't feel like they are being listened to and they are just being pushed out the door." In contrast to this, the volunteers at the clinic work to create a safe and welcoming environment.

This difference in Centro's approach to care is also demonstrated in the clinic's consideration (or really lack thereof) of the insurance and immigration status of their patients. In fact, the clinic's publicity and recruitment materials, website, and annual reports make no mention of the immigration status of the clinic's patients, though the majority of them are undocumented. A clinic volunteer administrator discussed the important difference of the de-emphasis on immigration and insurance status in comparison to mainstream health clinics: "We have an interesting way of doing business. We actually see people who do not have health insurance, sometimes those people don't have local IDs either. Too often, the funding agencies at the state and federal and government level require a certain level of documentation and identification that we just don't care about. We are here to deliver health services, and we could care less if someone has insurance or has the ID that the government or state might require." In this quote itself, even though she is discussing immigration status, the administrator does not explicitly call attention to this status. Rather, she reframes the issue as the problem of the requirements of documentation and identification, "issues" that are irrelevant within the clinic space except for the limitations that they foist on patients who cannot access care elsewhere.

In discussing Centro, clinic organizers describe their work and the organization as "a crucial component of Southern Arizona's medical infrastructure and health care system." Centro sees itself as helping those who have "fallen through the cracks" and "a safety net for the community," and rather than being separate from the mainstream health system, they argue that they are "integrating the private medical community" through donations and in-kind services for their patients. Central to the operation of the Third Net—and its vital position in relation to health care infrastructure—is this two-way "integration" of Third Net clinics and organizations with the mainstream medical community. On the one hand, Third Net spaces like Centro and the other organizations discussed in this chapter are reliant on the expertise of volunteer health care providers from the mainstream health system to care for their patients. At the same time, these health care providers bring with them connections to colleagues in the mainstream health system, which enables Third Net spaces to rely on informal and ad hoc networks of specialist care. For Centro, they describe the central importance of "selective referrals" to their health care provision. Because of their expansive networks within the mainstream health system, Centro volunteers are able to negotiate free care for things like mammograms and deep discounts on specialist care for their patients, and then Centro pays for these additional services, from lab work to surgery. In fact, because of these strong referral networks and discounted care, the clinic is able to provide its patients with more and more surgeries, in particular for hernias and cataracts. In one unique example, clinic volunteers networked with a hospital in California to get discounted hip replacement surgery for a 19-year-old patient with a large tumor on her hip. A core part of Centro's selective referrals also includes a long-time relationship with San Augustine's, a local Federally Qualified Health Center (FQHC) that provides primary and limited specialist care on a sliding scale to Tucson residents.[12] In this way, Centro is able to leverage their integration with the mainstream medical community to get preventative, primary, and specialist care that would otherwise be impossible for their patients to access. The challenges with these referrals come in the hours of logistical conversations with doctor's offices and hospital billing departments because often the "front desk and back desk are not in communication." As a result, Centro has a designated volunteer whose job is to coordinate with the billing departments to ensure the discounted rate of care for their patients.

As a free clinic, Centro as an organization and its volunteers intentionally structure the clinic offerings to approximate the health care options available to patients in the mainstream system, even if this means working through "selective referrals" to broker particular services, like surgery and some screenings, that Centro cannot offer in house. At the same time that it strives to be a traditional clinic for its patients, Centro works to cultivate a clinic space that is "different in all the right ways," meaning that the volunteers cultivate a philosophy of care that rectifies some of the shortcomings of the mainstream health system, including personalized care for their patients by volunteer providers committed to listening to them, taking their health concerns seriously, and working to "give back" to the community.

Charity in the Third Net

Closely aligned with the work and approach of a free clinic model, other organizations within the Third Net also provide free health services to uninsured, undocumented migrants but do so from an organizational framework that is more clearly defined as a charity. By "charity," we are referring to an organization that seeks to meet the immediate needs of people living in poverty through the provision of services performed for public benefit, rather than private interest or in the pursuit of profit.[13] The philosophy and organization of charity is inherently hierarchical, in which a benefactor provides a service or good for free (or at reduced cost) to a beneficiary. The beneficiary is deemed "needy" in some or multiple ways, and the benefactor, out of altruistic, moral, and/or financial motivation,[14] seeks to meet these needs, whether as a food bank handing out meals or a health care charity providing free medical services.

Unlike the history of free clinics detailed above, charity organizations invoke another history that is not entirely separate from the health care provision of free clinics, but that also encompasses a specific genealogy and approach to social service delivery. Charity has been the predominant mode of care for people living in poverty for centuries, and early poor relief measures in medieval Europe and later in the US were largely driven by religious individuals and organizations who believed they had a moral duty to perform charitable acts or give alms to the poor.[15] Many charitable organizations continue to operate with overtly religious missions to provide social services like food, housing, education, and health care that are not (or are no longer) provided through government programs.

Charity organizations in the Third Net draw their roots largely from the public almshouses (or "poorhouses") and the "free medical dispensaries" of the late 18th and 19th centuries. Almshouses served as catch-all institutions for housing not only destitute children, widows, and the elderly but also impoverished people with substance use issues, disabilities, contagious diseases, mental health issues, and long-term health conditions that necessitated care. An examination of almshouses in New York City from the 1930s found that one in five residents needed health care and a quarter of these ill residents were bed-ridden from their health issues.[16] In many ways, after the Social Security Act, these early almshouses birthed the public hospital as we know it today, but they also continue their legacy in the charity organizations that provide health care for uninsured and underinsured patients across the US.[17] A lesser-known health-related charity during these times was the free public dispensary, which was likened to a "medical soup kitchen" and primarily distributed free medications to indigent patients.[18] Dispensaries also operated as small community-based health facilities where medical students practiced diagnosing and treating patients as a way to further their medical education.[19] As neoliberal austerity measures have continued to erode the few social welfare programs in the US over the past decades, the sector of charity organizations working to meet people's basic needs has grown into a multi-billion-dollar industry.

Within health care provision, "charity" has a variety of related implications. This traditional understanding of charity as working to meet the needs of people living in poverty has given rise to the notion of "charity care." Charity care specifically refers to the provision of free or low-cost medical care to someone who is without insurance and/or cannot afford to pay their health care costs. Charity care is part and parcel of the mainstream health system and safety net in the US, through which physicians and other medical providers offer pro bono health care to indigent patients. Charity care has also grown to encompass patients on Medicaid and the work of public hospitals that provide care to these patients. In this way, charity care is firmly ensconced in health care provision within the overall health system and safety net, although it is certainly related to the work of the Third Net.

Although there are significant overlaps, the charity model of health care in the Third Net is distinct from that of free clinics. Within the "traditional" organizational model, these philosophies of care both assume a needs-based (rather than a rights-based) approach to health care provision. As outlined in table 1.2, they share similar funding structures and formalized referral networks. However, the distinction between these approaches rests largely on their organizational infrastructure, which shapes the way the organizations frame their mission, vision, and approach to patients and donors. In free clinics, the relationship between volunteers and patients is one that largely mirrors that of the patient-provider relationship in the mainstream health system, whereas charities maintain a benefactor-beneficiary relationship that is well established in many poor relief programs. The emphasis is on the deservingness of their beneficiaries and is made evident through framing stories of patients' gratitude and exemplary work ethic. Within the Third Net, traditional charity organizations, like Grace in Action, draw from this legacy of religious-based charity health work to meet the immediate, pressing medical needs of uninsured, undocumented migrants.

Grace in Action: A Religious Charity's Healing through the Power of Love

As the only fully mobile, free health care organization in Phoenix, Grace in Action (informally, Grace) hosts clinic days five days a week at seven different church locations across the Phoenix metro area. On clinic days, the organization's huge RV, retrofitted as a mobile clinic space and pharmacy, travels to each of the churches to provide primary health care and free prescription services to "the uninsured working poor and homeless of all ages" across the city. The clinics are run out of large church auditoriums that look like they could host a theater production or a basketball rec tournament. Instead, on clinic days, they are filled with tables and folding chairs and boxes upon boxes of patient files in the makeshift check-in and waiting room area. As the start of the clinic nears, a long line of patients snakes outside the door. When patients are called for their appointment, they are led to one of about 30 tables throughout the middle of the open auditorium, where a volunteer health provider awaits their next patient. Many of these volunteers are older retired doctors and nurses volunteering their time and expertise to "give back" through the work and mission of Grace.

With an overtly religious organizational approach, Grace works to "restore dignity" for uninsured and underinsured patients who can't afford health care or prescriptions in the mainstream health system. Part of Grace's mission is to implement "healing through love" by providing free health care. Although some of the clinic's residents are undocumented migrants, the organization does not discuss their immigration status explicitly in their promotional materials. However, in addition to being used for clinic spaces due to the religious nature of the organization, churches are also trusted safe spaces for undocumented migrants, one of the only "sacred" spaces where Immigration and Custom Enforcement (ICE) does not conduct raids.[20] This perception of safety is particularly important in Phoenix, where former Sheriff Arpaio's workplace and community raids created a real culture of fear among migrant communities in the metro area. This culture of fear, which caused parents to keep their kids out of school and made residents hesitant to drive or ride the bus around town, also hindered migrants' ability to access health care in mainstream medical spaces and put additional pressures on Third Net organizations to provide this care in trusted and safe environments.[21]

In operation for almost 25 years, Grace is the largest and most well-resourced of all the organizations in our study, serving almost 3,000 patients across the Phoenix metro area. The majority of these patients (80%) when they first come to Grace have undiagnosed and untreated health conditions such as hypertension, high cholesterol, and diabetes. Although these are manageable conditions, the patients at Grace are unable to afford to see the doctor or pay for their medications. Grace works to provide a "continuum of care" beyond emergency services or health screenings so that their patients can have a "medical home" and a regular primary care physician. For Grace, as for so many other Third Net organizations, regular preventative and primary care is critical to its ability to care for its patients by avoiding more serious medical needs, such as insulin dependence, that quickly become prohibitively expensive for both the patients and the organization providing them care. By offering preventative and regular primary care, Grace helps patients "avoid dangerous complications and costly emergency care."

Grace's other main service is the large number of free prescriptions it offers its patients, with over 225 generic prescription medications, to help patients navigate and manage their health conditions. Without these free medications, patients would not otherwise be able to afford the necessary prescriptions. In its promotional materials, Grace discusses the central importance of offering free medication to their patients so that they can "maintain their health [which allows] them to return to work, care for their family, or resume productive lives."

Like other Third Net organizations, Grace is reliant on its own relationships and networks for patient referrals to additional pro bono and reduced-cost care that the organization itself cannot provide. To formalize these largely ad hoc relationships, Grace operates a "Compassionate Community Partners" network, which is a referral network to doctors and hospitals across the Phoenix metro area who have agreed to provide care to Grace's patients that are referred directly from the organization.

Grace provides an important case of Third Net organizations for a variety of reasons: 1) it operates as a partially mobile clinic, 2) it has a religious-based mission, and 3) it models itself as a traditional charity organization. Migrant health care in the US has a long history of using mobile health clinics (MHCs) to reach migrant patients, primarily agricultural workers, who are otherwise unable to access health care. Usually, MHCs operate independently from brick-and-mortar clinic structures and travel to fields or other areas where migrants are working or to communities where they are living. Additionally, they often do not operate strict hours for appointments so that workers can access care on demand and outside of their usual working hours. As an important aspect of migrant health across the US, MHCs usually provide care in more rural areas of the country where migrant workers have even less access to health care options. In some ways, then, Grace does not fit this particular model of MHCs, as it offers more of an urban, hybrid option between mobile and fixed clinic sites. Although it has an RV specially outfitted for patient screenings and prescription medication distribution, the mobile unit itself travels from church to church across the metro area and operates at specific daytime hours each week on an appointment, rather than drop-in, basis. The mobile unit complements the rotating yet fixed brick-and-mortar clinic spaces in church auditoriums across Phoenix.

Furthermore, Grace operates as an explicitly religious organization drawing from a long history of faith-based health and humanitarian aid nonprofit organizations and charities working nationally and internationally to support migrants and refugees. Encouraged by its Christian values, the organization is composed of volunteers who not only are working to give back to their communities (like the primary altruistic motivations of volunteers at clinics like Centro), but are also motivated specifically by a religious imperative to care for the "foreigners" and the poor within their midst. Grace's religious mission to restore dignity to its indigent patients is similar to that of the early public dispensaries. In many ways, it would not be disingenuous to liken Grace to a "medical soup kitchen" in which the organization focuses on maximizing the number of patient visits they have each year as well as the thousands of dollars of in-kind, free prescription medications that they are able to distribute to these patients to manage their chronic health conditions.

Social Justice Organizations in the Third Net

Whereas Centro de Salud and Grace in Action are representative of more "traditional" approaches to migrant health, the next two organizations illustrate a free clinic and a charity premised on a more explicitly social justice mission and vision. Social justice as a philosophy of care represents a considerable portion of the organizations, nonprofits, and clinic spaces in the Third Net who are not only working to provide health care services to meet the immediate needs of their patients, but are also allocating attention, time, effort, and resources to recognizing the larger structural issues giving rise to migrants' ineligibility for care and their experiences of health disparities.

This philosophy of care involves both a discourse and a practice around migrant health. Often, social justice organizations approach their missions from a rights-based perspective, rather than the needs-based approach of traditional charity organizations. It involves the discursive framing of health as a human right for all regardless of income or immigration status.[22] This fundamental recognition of health as a human right often leads social justice organizations to critique the failures of the current health system and the larger sociopolitical structure of the US to guarantee health care access and provision for all. Beyond the exclusion of migrants from insurance coverage and health access, they also indict the US immigration system and the punitive enforcement tactics that discourage migrants from accessing what few social services to which they remain entitled, including seeking emergency health care in the mainstream system.[23] Further, the discursive strategies of Third Net social justice organizations, which will be discussed in more detail in later chapters, also include reframing the anti-immigrant rhetoric of undeservingness and exclusion that figures migrants as burdens or as "illegals."

The medical provision and work of social justice organizations is essentially health activism in practice, directly challenging migrants' exclusion from health care.[24] These organizations pay attention to the factors that contribute to migrants' disenfranchisement, including health and immigration policies and immigration enforcement tactics of detention and deportation, and they often work to educate their volunteers and communities about these policies and practices. Beyond direct health provision, then, they also work to foster systemic and social change on micro and/or macro levels, including social movement activity like protests, political advocacy, electoral work, and direct action.

The next two Third Net organizations adopt a social justice philosophy of care that is rooted in migrant rights, health justice, and Catholic worker movements: a free clinic (CommUnity Clinic of Phoenix) and a charity organization (Justicia y Paz).

CommUnity Clinic of Phoenix: Social Justice in a Free Clinic

Run out of a small house, CommUnity Clinic of Phoenix (informally, either CommUnity or CCP) is a free clinic for uninsured, undocumented patients. There is no sign outside the clinic or any other indication that the building is anything other than a residential home. Before it was a clinic, the house had been condemned because it had fallen into disrepair after being owned by someone who hoarded animals and was also operating as the neighborhood "crack house" for using and procuring illicit drugs. The house was sold by the city with the expectation that the buyer would tear it down and develop the large lot. Instead, CCP volunteers Ed and Donna bought it, gutted the building, and remodeled it as a house that could also be used as a clinic space. Michael, one of CCP's main nursing volunteers, reminisced, "Before we had the clinic, we were just doing house calls and seeing patients out of the kitchen at the local immigrant rights center." He motioned around him to the tiny kitchen-turned-volunteer-office with floor-to-ceiling shelves of medical supplies: "It's cramped quarters here for sure, but it's drastically increased our capacity to see patients. Ed likes to joke that it's just a different kind of drug house now."

The clinic's 500 patients mostly deal with treatable chronic health issues such as diabetes, hypertension, high cholesterol, and/or thyroid issues, but because they do not have insurance or authorized immigration status, these health conditions have usually gone undiagnosed and untreated for years. In addition to providing primary care services, CommUnity also provides some limited specialist care, such as midwifery and physical therapy, depending on the expertise of the current volunteers. CommUnity also partnered with a local naturopathic medical school in the Phoenix area, so naturopathic volunteers work with patients to offer homeopathic treatments. Holistic health volunteers, including a local curandera, offer healing work with crystals and feathers as well as limited mental health support through mindfulness and talk therapy. The clinic operates two days a week, and volunteers also still make house calls to patients throughout the week, monitoring the health of the most acute patients and those with transportation issues that keep them from the clinic.

The clinic relies on hundreds of volunteers to provide a variety of primary and specialist care, fundraise, clean the clinic, restock medical supplies, and generally keep the organization running. The volunteers include an interesting mix of people: members of a street medic collective (original founders of the clinic) that provides health care at migrant rights protests; doctors, nurses, and physician assistants working in local hospitals and medical offices; curanderas and other spiritual healers who are themselves migrants; and young, affluent white suburbanites who are aspiring medical students looking for experience with "underserved populations." The clinic founders assert that the organization has always been "unapologetically activist" in its approach to health care for those who they describe in their official mission as the "medically-marginalized."

In contrast to traditional free clinics, CommUnity frames its work as aligned with social justice principles. Its unofficial mission stresses that the organization is "not a free version of a broken system." In other words, rather than replicating a traditional clinic space within the Third Net, CCP works to create a free clinic that intentionally challenges the shortcomings of the mainstream health system.[25] Through their volunteer trainings and public-facing media presence, clinic volunteers critique the "brokenness" of the US health care and immigration systems, while working to effect social change, especially on the local and state levels. They also view their health care provision for uninsured, undocumented migrants within the larger anti-immigrant environment of Phoenix as health activism.[26]

In Phoenix, there are virtually no formal avenues for uninsured, undocumented migrants to access care in the mainstream health system. Additionally, anti-immigrant rhetoric and legislation has translated into punitive immigration enforcement that dampens migrants' health-seeking behavior. However, in this inhospitable environment for migrants, CCP volunteers use their expertise and prestige as medical professionals (who largely work in formal health settings for their day jobs) and their networks of colleagues to broker care for their patients through informal channels into the mainstream health system. For instance, CCP volunteers use their networks to negotiate pro bono specialist care for some of their patients in need of more complex medical procedures, from biopsies to heart surgery. In other examples, CommUnity organizes crowd-funding campaigns for patients in need of costly procedures and care that the clinic itself cannot provide. For example, they raised over $40,000 to pay for discounted surgery for Yolie, a single mom with young children, who crushed her arm when she fell off a ladder. After the many pins were removed from her arm post-surgery, she was able to get the rehabilitation she needed at no cost from CCP's volunteer physical therapist. As important as this informal or semi-formal brokerage is for individual patients, this model of brokerage for all five hundred of the clinic's patients would be unsustainable and unrealistic. As a result, brokerage into the mainstream health system negotiated by CCP volunteers only occurs on an individualized, ad hoc, and case-by-case basis, using sometimes unorthodox methods between the Third Net and the formal health system.

Part of the social justice mission of the organization involves a refiguring of the role of migrants—both within the wider Phoenix community and in the clinic itself. Challenging the ideas of migrants as "burdens" or drains on collective resources, Donna, one of the main clinic founders and core organizers, asserts,

> Around the country, but particularly in Arizona, we see anti-immigrant rhetoric that portrays immigrants as burdens. This is especially true in discussions about health care, as if immigrants don't deserve to go to the doctor. This rhetoric shows up in harsh immigration policies like SB1070 [the infamous Arizona legislation that allows local police to check the immigration status of anyone they arrest or detain] . . . but it's important to recognize that it's not immigrants that are the burden. It's the denial of health care, not uninsured immigrants, that is a burden on society as a whole.

In this discussion, Donna challenges the anti-immigrant rhetoric that frames migrants as "burdensome non-patients" and promotes a framework which sees migrants as "patients within a burdensome system." Adopting a larger structural critique, Donna emphasizes the ways that policies like SB1070 create situations in which migrants are racialized as "illegal" and burdensome. Health care legislation that denies migrants health coverage and access to medical services plays a significant role in the construction of migrants as encumbering the system, emphasizing the costs that they incur rather than their contributions to society. CommUnity works to frame migrants at the clinic first and foremost as *patients*, emphasizing their right to health care access and provision. The problem then for CCP is with a larger system that refuses to recognize the patient status of uninsured migrants and actively works to deny them health care coverage and services.

In addition to challenging the portrayal of migrants as burdens in anti-immigrant rhetoric, CCP also reframes the traditional clinical hierarchies of patient-provider relationships. Part of the organization's vision is to manifest a larger CCP community where patients fight for their own rights to health care. Their understanding of migrants as patients is a far cry from many clinics, including Centro de Salud, in which the role patients occupy is one in which they are solely on the receiving end of services. First and foremost, CCP emphasizes the fact that the clinic's patients are members of the same larger community, and the language most often used regarding patients at the clinic is that of "neighbor." Consistently across fundraising appeals and social media posts, this image of a community of neighbors is central, emphasizing a mutuality, rather than a hierarchical relationship, between patients and providers, between citizens and noncitizens. This vision is emphasized in one of CCP's funding letters, saying, "Together, we really can build a better world, where all our neighbors, regardless of immigration status, know that their lives and health are valued." In this way, CCP challenges anti-immigrant rhetoric of dependency by highlighting migrants' right to belonging and health as neighbors, while indicting the US health care system for denying migrants' right to health care.

Migrants at CCP also play an active role in organizational activities. In addition to understanding patients and volunteers as "neighbors" in the same larger community, CCP volunteers recognize patients not as passive recipients of health care or other social services but, rather, as active organizers working to claim their own rights. For instance, in a volunteer training session, Michael, a nurse and CCP volunteer, said,

> What you have to know is that our patients are part of a very strong and very organized immigrant community in this state. They are by no means drains on the system, and at the same time, they are by no means victims that are taking this sitting down. They are gutsy and smart organizers fighting for their own rights.

By describing patients as both neighbors within a larger health community and organizers fighting for their own rights, CCP volunteers explicitly recognize migrants' active role in facilitating their health care. This recognition disrupts traditional patient-provider configurations and opens possibilities for migrants to serve as brokers themselves.

At CommUnity, migrants are not only among the patients, but also volunteer as medical professionals and caregivers at the clinic. For example, Octavia, a migrant herself, provides patients talk therapy and mindfulness exercises to help alleviate stress and anxiety. Javiera, a migrant and volunteer from the Hispanic Nurses' Association, not only provides care at CCP but also uses the space to educate current and future medical professionals about the challenges faced by uninsured, undocumented migrants in the US, like her parents and brother: "Before coming here, I didn't know that clinics like this existed. Now I can't see myself ever not working in a clinic like CCP."

CommUnity recognizes that not all new volunteers know or fully understand the relationship between the organization's anti-racist and health justice aims. Clinic volunteers represent a diverse mix of people from across spectrums of age, race, immigration status, citizenship, and socioeconomic status. This diversity of volunteers comes with a particular set of challenges around fostering the mission of the organization, including providing equitable health care with cultural humility and establishing a non-hierarchical, collaborative environment. The early clinic volunteers came largely from within the migrant rights movement in Phoenix and already had a robust knowledge of the anti-immigrant sentiment and structural challenges faced by the clinic's patients. However, as the clinic became more established, it attracted a cohort of volunteers— mostly white, affluent, suburban young adults. Lorena, one of the original founders of the clinic, discussed this influx of new volunteers:

> We end up getting a lot of white, suburban kids as volunteers who want to go into medicine. With PA [physician assistant] school being so competitive, their applications are more likely to get a look with them having volunteered with "underserved" communities. But they come to us without the knowledge of immigrant rights or health justice, and this means that we have to go through a process of educating them about what our patients are up against. Otherwise, we end up replicating the power inequalities of patient-provider relationships . . . and, in this context, that looks a lot like white saviorism.

Destabilizing the larger racial dynamics and power inequalities of patient-provider interactions demands vigilance and intentionality. Educating new volunteers is a core activity of the clinic, which hosts regular volunteer orientations and trainings on things like immigration policy and health justice so that new volunteers understand the larger social and political context in which the clinic's patients must survive. In this way, CCP volunteers work to inform the knowledge and perspectives of future medical professionals and hopefully shape their future medical provision. This education also involves, at least implicitly, a challenge to traditional systems of brokerage and hierarchies of patient-provider relationships.

Although it shares many of the same health care services as Centro, CommUnity frames its mission in a way that is explicitly social justice oriented, meaning that it stresses a rights-based approach to migrant health care and educates its volunteers in ways that challenge the rhetoric around the undeservingness of migrant patients as well as the power hierarchies of traditional patient-provider relationships. This social justice model is also evident in its local advocacy on migrant rights and health justice so that the clinic volunteers work to meet the immediate health needs of their patients, while promoting systemic change to the anti-immigrant policies that directly affect their patients' access to health care and other social services.

Justicia y Paz: A Religious Social Justice Charity

Situated in the middle of one of Harris County's rapidly developing neighborhoods, Justicia y Paz (informally, Justicia) is a faith-based non-governmental organization in Houston, Texas, that provides free basic medical care, food, clothing, and temporary shelter to hundreds of low-income undocumented migrants each year. Structurally, Justicia is separated into a "women's house" and a "men's house"—two buildings that sit back-to-back on the same neighborhood block. Children, female volunteers, and migrant women reside in the former. Male volunteers and migrant men reside in the latter. While the women's house is two stories tall and can house up to 40 people, the men's house is wide and can provide shelter for up to 65 people. Since its initiation in 1980, Justicia has run exclusively on volunteer labor and donations from communities and parishes across the world, including the Vatican. It has never received government funding. Like other spaces inspired by the Catholic Worker Movement,[27] Justicia operates with the philosophy that since the state is ill equipped to meet the needs of the poor, it must serve as a "house of hospitality" for the region's undocumented population. This means that Justicia volunteers (referred to as "Catholic Workers") treat every undocumented migrant who comes to its doors as a Christlike figure whose needs should be actively attended to, regardless of how big or small these needs are.

Conceptualizing care in both medical and non-medical terms, Justicia facilitates a range of free activities and services, including but not limited to 1) recruiting volunteer doctors from Houston's medical district to provide primary health care services to nearly 300 undocumented migrants each month, 2) offering financial support to over 100 migrant families in need of home health care assistance, 3) helping migrants navigate formal medical bureaucracies, and 4) providing temporary gender-segregated shelter. Additional services include coordination with other community organizations, weekly food and clothing distributions, daily delivery of brown-bagged lunches to day laborers and the homeless, and bi-weekly ESL courses for the organization's migrant "guests." In line with the Catholic Worker Movement, the combination of these activities is intended to synergize charity and social justice frameworks to accomplish the goals of meeting migrants' needs.

In localities like Houston, Texas, formal initiatives like the annually renewable Harris Health financial assistance program—also known as the Gold Card—offer up to 100% coverage for medical expenses incurred within the Harris Health System (informally, Harris Health).[28] To qualify, individuals must present proof of income, residency, and identity; legal status is not a concern. Accordingly, Justicia volunteers do everything they can to help migrants obtain these proofs and become eligible for the Gold Card. In fact, Harris Health accepts a signed form from Justicia as proof of income and residency, though Justicia residents often struggle to get a valid ID to complete their Gold Card application.[29] Assuming migrants have some form of identification, Justicia can help undocumented migrants become formally eligible for health coverage otherwise federally denied to them, effectively facilitating their way into the First and Second Nets of the health care system.

Justicia asserts that entitlement to health care is actually based on a higher-level spiritual law that recognizes migrants' humanity. According to Margaret, one of the founding co-directors, this sentiment reflects the Bible's "Sermon on the Mount" in Matthew 25 in which Jesus Christ instructs people to care for the poor as they would care for him: "What you do for the least of the brethren you do for me." Every volunteer references this verse when explaining their motivation for joining the group, and according to Margaret, Matthew 25 captures the whole essence of the organization's mission and aims. Laurie, a volunteer, shares that whenever anyone asks Margaret how they can ever repay Justicia for its support, Margaret always makes some reference to the passage or simply responds "Matthew 25," suggesting that people can repay Justicia by providing whatever support they can to others. For volunteers (i.e., Catholic Workers), this directive supersedes health and immigration laws that might limit or prevent practitioners from providing care to low-income undocumented migrants. In an article published six years into Justicia's ongoing 40-year existence, Larry (the organization's co-director) explained,

> At [Justicia y Paz], we don't worry about breaking the law. In fact, we are totally distracted by trying to keep the law, the Law of the Gospels, that says that we must love our neighbors as ourselves. Rejecting homeless people, refugees, mothers and children because they don't have I.D. is like rejecting Jesus. True, we may be too fundamentalist or literal in our interpretation of Matthew 25, but then we are stuck with being Catholic Workers.

Several volunteers echo Larry's sentiment and conclude that rejecting "the poor" is like rejecting Christ himself. Rather than concern themselves with immigration and health care laws, Catholic Workers focus solely on upholding the "Law of the Gospels," which do not require documentation. Larry succinctly captures this sentiment: "We haven't met an illegal alien in our six years as Justicia y Paz. We have met a lot of people, though." Here, illegality signifies racialized disentitlement and less-than-human status. In replacing the notion of "illegal aliens" with "people," Larry and other Catholic Workers challenge the prohibitive and dehumanizing connotations of illegality and emphasize migrants' humanity. Expressions of humanity like this are important to and common among the organization's volunteers. For example, when Consuelo, a volunteer, was asked what she hopes migrants will remember from their time at Justicia, she responded: "That in [Justicia y Paz], they were treated like human beings."

At Justicia, volunteers do what they can to decenter their role as brokers, but this can be challenging. Victoria, a volunteer, provides an example, explaining a moment when she took a migrant woman named Brenda to an appointment in Houston's medical district:

> When you're with someone [at a hospital] and it's about them and their life and their situation, and then the professional talks to [me], I'm like,

Brenda's right here, and she understands you; speaks English . . . It's not me. It's not my medical problem [or] legal problem. It's not my anything. Like, I just drove Brenda here . . . I'm not her social worker.

Victoria expresses frustration with becoming the center of attention among health practitioners and emphasizes that the clinic visit is about Brenda. In doing so, Victoria tries to decenter the broker role and re-center Brenda in the health care interaction. In emphasizing that she is not Brenda's social worker, Victoria rejects the conventional liaison role of health care brokers and expresses desire for a relationship where she is peripheral, rather than central, to addressing Brenda's health care needs.

This was a common experience among a predominately white base of volunteers at Justicia. Health practitioners routinely asked volunteers questions about migrants' health even though these migrants were sitting in the same room, perfectly capable of articulating their own needs. Victoria reflects on these experiences:

> I feel weird about it. I don't know what it is. Is it the language? Is it race? Is it both those things? I don't know, but it does frustrate me, and I struggle a lot with the idea of the white savior complex and [whether or not] I'm perpetuating it by being here.

Brokerage processes are generally understood in practical "means-to-an-end" terms (i.e., the job of the broker is to facilitate access to care), but here, Victoria illustrates deeper considerations about what it means to be a broker. In this Third Net context, brokerage also means challenging the conditions that make brokering care necessary in the first place. In other words, Victoria and other volunteers want to make themselves (i.e., the broker role) unnecessary or irrelevant. Doing so, however, requires critical evaluation of the health and immigration policies that structure migrants' experiences of exclusion and affirm hierarchical brokerage relations.

Within Justicia, hierarchies of migrant-volunteer relationships that are evident in traditional charities like Grace are challenged and destabilized, and migrants are empowered to take on leadership roles within the organization. One Catholic Worker, Carolina, is a migrant herself and conducts medical intake at the clinic every week. Her family received medical care from Justicia several years prior to her arrival in the country, and now she has been providing this care herself for about six years: "It's so funny. In the beginning, Margaret didn't even want me to touch the computer. She was like, 'don't touch anything; just watch!' And now I'm like in charge of the clinic [*laughs*]." Studying to be a physician assistant, Carolina occupies a leadership role in the clinic. When other volunteers have questions about clinic protocol, they commonly turn to Carolina.

In many cases, migrants join volunteers at Justicia in a range of activities, including weekly food distributions, cooking and cleaning, and caregiving. In turn, they too become brokers of care. Like volunteers, migrants help one another fill out Gold Card (i.e., financial assistance) applications, share information about reliable clinics, and provide linguistic assistance during medical visits. This is particularly important for migrants like 46-year-old Joseph, who suffered a debilitating car accident and speaks in low mumbles. Elias, a 75-year-old Mexican man, is among a select few who are able to understand Joseph. Accordingly, Elias makes sure Joseph takes his medicine every day and routinely accompanies Joseph to medical appointments outside of Justicia in order to literally speak on his behalf. The Third Net's informality allows for a renegotiation of roles such that Joseph, a migrant who also needs care (conventionally the "patient"), can act as both caregiver (health practitioner) and care facilitator (broker).

The case of Justicia demonstrates the ways that social justice–oriented organizations not only meet immediate needs of migrants—whether health-related or other material needs—but also work to envision new relationships and configurations of care. For Justicia, these new configurations rely on a faith-based vision in which marginalized people are welcomed and cared for outside of the parameters of the state. In this vision, migrants are not just beneficiaries of care but active participants.

For both CommUnity and Justicia, social justice principles, related to the position of migrants within their communities and the fundamental right to health for everyone, serve as the foundation for these organizations' framing of their work and health care provision to migrants. For CommUnity, this social justice foundation influences the way that the organization tries to model a free clinic that does not replicate the brokenness of the mainstream health system, while for Justicia, this religiously motivated social justice mission involves visioning inclusion and belonging for migrants beyond the policies and programs of the State. Together, these examples demonstrate organizations premised on a philosophy of care that is explicitly oriented toward social justice. For CommUnity, immigration and health care laws are inherently problematic, and for Justicia, these laws are inferior to the "Law of the Gospels." Despite being oriented by different ideologies, practitioners within both organizations recognize the structural constraints of the US health care system and seek to do more than simply facilitate migrants' access to it. For volunteers in both spaces, brokerage also involves status-shifting.[30] CommUnity volunteers attempt to shift migrants' status from "burdensome non-patients" to "patients within a burdensome system," and Justicia volunteers try to shift migrants' status from "illegal aliens" to "human beings" with real needs and capabilities.

As a result, both organizations wrestle with realizing their social justice visions within the current constraints of health and immigration policy in the US. Part of this work involves looking inward as organizations to challenge and re-vision patient-provider relationships within the clinic spaces, while other aspects of this work involve leveraging their reputations and influence to shape the health care access and experiences of migrants in their communities.

Mutual Aid as a Philosophy of Care

Another philosophy of care within the Third Net in the US is mutual aid, a framework that has gained more general popularity and traction in recent times of crisis, including through community-based responses to natural disasters and social crises like the COVID-19 pandemic. Mutual aid is a cooperative framework based on the reciprocal exchange of goods, skills, ideas, and other resources often between members of the same community or individuals in similar social groups. Mutual aid is premised on the idea that everyone has something they can contribute, and everyone has something they need. As Mariame Kaba described it, "It's not community service—you're not doing service for service's sake. You're trying to address real material needs."[31] In addition to addressing material needs, mutual aid is also based on solidarity in a struggle against a common challenge or in efforts to leverage and create systemic change. Dean Spade defines mutual aid as "a form of political participation in which people take responsibility for caring for one another and changing political conditions, not just through symbolic acts or putting pressure on their representatives in government but by actually building new social relations that are more survivable."[32]

Before mutual aid's newfound popularity, it had been used for centuries among Indigenous groups, labor organizations, African Americans or "free blacks," civil rights groups like the Black Panthers, and migrant groups in the US. From the late 1700s to late 1800s, "mutual benefit societies" of "free blacks" in the US provided health and life insurance for newly arrived African Americans, free blacks, and fugitive slaves, focusing primarily on health care but also providing economic and social support and education.[33] In the late 1800s and early 1900s, "fraternal societies" organized and run by poor and working-class people provided mutual aid in the absence of social welfare programs, and primarily focused on medical aid. An 1894 report about these societies in New Hampshire noted, "The tendency to join fraternal organizations for the purpose of obtaining care and relief in the event of sickness is well-nigh universal."[34] These fraternal organizations were financed by monthly dues from members, who then created committees that decided how these funds would be allocated. The membership elected doctors that staffed the hospitals that the organizations had created and coordinated.[35] Especially during the influenza and yellow fever epidemics, fraternal societies organized health centers to care for their members. In addition to medical provision, the societies also offered access to paid sick leave and life insurance.

In many ways, mutual aid as a framework of community solidarity stands in direct opposition to traditional forms of charity and even against the prevailing hierarchies of social justice organizations.[36] According to Spade and others, mutual aid distinguishes itself from charity in fundamental and significant ways: it focuses on addressing basic needs while building solidarity and understanding of the root causes of inequity and then organizing to address these root causes through direct participation and collective action.[37] In this way, mutual aid as a philosophy of care flattens power hierarchies, in a direct response to and reaction against forms of charity that, at best, do not address the root causes of poverty in the US and, at worst, serve to prop up the current inequitable system and control poor people.

Drawing from the historical provision of health care and basic survival needs of mutual aid networks, a migrant rights organization in Harris County has been providing care among a group of undocumented migrants with disabilities in the Houston area.

Houston Health Action: Building Solidarity from the Margins through Mutual Aid

Houston Health Action (informally, Health Action or HHA) is a grassroots community-based, migrant-led organization of uninsured, undocumented migrants with disabilities, the majority of whom have experienced debilitating injuries or amputations. For nearly two decades, Health Action has worked to "affirm the dignity and improve the quality of life of migrants and refugees with disabilities and their families." Unlike the other Third Net organizations in our study, Health Action provides services to a subset of migrants with specific medical needs, primarily people with spinal cord injuries who use wheelchairs for mobility. Health Action describes its members as exploited and doubly marginalized as undocumented and disabled migrants.

In 2005, the Harris County Hospital District in Houston made the decision to stop providing medical supplies and services to people with spinal cord injuries who were not eligible for Medicaid. The medical conditions of these patients meant that their lives depended on vital medical supplies, including sterile catheters, diapers, urine drainage bags, and gloves. Out of pocket, these supplies would cost at least $400 a month, which is prohibitively expensive. These patients are virtually destitute as they are not eligible for public benefits, are uninsured, and are unable to work and so do not have a stable income. As a result, they struggle to access basic medical supplies and services that they need to survive. A small group of people directly affected by the Hospital District's decision banded together to create Health Action. Since then, they have worked tirelessly to "improve access to services, promote inclusion of people with disabilities, foster independence, enhance mobility, and demand equality."

One primary aim of the organization is to support each other to survive by collectively working to get the necessary resources, medical supplies, and equipment. The members fundraise for these medical supplies and supply them to all Health Action members. In the organization's initial years, these fundraising efforts included holding car washes and selling roses on street corners and at intersections across Houston. They also collected donated items, like TVs and small appliances, which they raffled off. More recently, the fundraising includes individual donations from people who support HHA's work. With this money, Health Action members buy the necessary supplies in bulk and then divide them among the organization's membership, which now numbers close to 200 people, through a monthly supply distribution. In this work, HHA is committed to "never leaving anyone behind" and ensuring that "no one leaves with their hands empty," as one of the members described it. In addition to providing these necessary medical supplies, members of the organization accept donations of used medical equipment, including wheelchairs, hospital beds, and shower chairs, then clean and fix them up before passing them on to the organization's members.

Beyond providing medical supplies and equipment, Health Action aims to foster hope and solidarity as an organization in order to improve the mental health and overall quality of life of its members. Its members work to combat isolation by building a support network, where people with similar experiences and challenges "can feel included, respected, and loved." The organization works to foster independence and autonomy for its members, yet at the same time create an intentional community of members that feels more like a chosen family. They share holiday celebrations, baby showers, birthday parties, even funerals. Health Action members collectively support each other through the traumas that they have survived and work to cultivate a community of members who "also support one another to heal, to grow and to educate others on how to deal with the physical and emotional challenges they face and the challenges that arise from navigating institutions and systems that perpetuate exclusion and resist equity." As part of this initiative, Health Action also operates a committee called the "Quality of Life Promoters." This committee receives word-of-mouth referrals from members of the organization, the wider community, and even hospitals and social service agencies. Quality of Life Promoters visit people in hospitals and their homes in the early days after their health crises to support them through the initial trauma of their injuries, educate them about the practicalities of living with a spinal cord injury, invite them to engage with Health Action and its activities, and also advise them on their rights as an undocumented person with disabilities. Much of the solidarity and quality of life support that Health Action members provide to each other intentionally combats isolation and mental health struggles.

In addition to meeting each other's day-to-day medical and emotional needs, Health Action strategically works to build collective leadership among the organization's members so that they can engage in community advocacy efforts. An HHA report provides a scathing indictment of the situation in which its members are forced to live, and motivates the members and the organization to fight for change. "We have seen people living in terrible conditions not due to a lack of resources in our society, but due to the callous insensitivity of those in power at the federal and state level and the pervasive inequality in access to resources and opportunities." In their work of leadership development, Health Action intentionally centers the experiences of people who are multiply marginalized and supports them as leaders and advocates for themselves and others like them who are left behind and excluded. These leaders then engage in advocacy efforts built on a framework that draws from principles of disability rights, health justice, and migrant rights. Their advocacy efforts have included everything from stopping a fare increase for public transportation in Harris County to lobbying against anti-immigrant legislation at the state level.

In all its efforts, HHA is not only working to highlight the exclusion and exploitation of its members but also their strength and resilience. Health Action describes its overall efforts saying, "We are highlighting vulnerability, marginalization and discrimination, but we are also telling the stories of solidarity, resilience and hope that keep our communities going." In this way, its members are not only diagnosing the current failures of the system that negatively affect them, but also envisioning a better world and working to realize the changes necessary to achieve it. Fundamental to this vision is a society in which "migrants, people with disabilities and poor people [are] seen as being an integral part of our society. Health systems, hospitals, schools should not frame these constituencies as burdens to solve. Policymakers and elected officials should also start seeing and talking about these constituencies as important part of our society and communities. Only then can we begin to look at challenges holistically in order to solve them." In this vision set out by Health Action, its members who are marginalized in multiple ways have a seat at the table and a say in decisions that are made about themselves and their communities. HHA reimagines a society in which the most marginalized—people with disabilities, undocumented migrants, and others—are at the center of planning and policymaking and are "there from the beginning and not an afterthought."[38]

HHA members work to realize this vision of a society that centers the voices and experiences of undocumented migrants with disabilities through an infrastructure built on the distribution of life-saving supplies, the solidarity that they foster, and the advocacy efforts through which they affect positive change for not only their members but the larger community in which they live. They challenge the notion that other people can speak for their needs. "For the most part, there is no such thing as being the voice of the voiceless and what is needed is an increased capacity of institutions to actually listen and respond to what communities are saying." This vision and work are fundamentally built on the foundation and framework of mutual aid.

"Mutual aid" generally refers to networks of support and reciprocity that work together to meet collective needs through sharing resources and organizing on a community level. Health Action members describe the mutual aid work of the organization as fundamentally "sharing what we have and organizing to get what we need." In many ways, the mutual aid framework of Health Action is antithetical to traditional charity models, in that it is centered on a reciprocal relationship among the organization's members. One volunteer described it in this way: "I see this organization as a net that is able to catch and to sustain our own community."[39] Through this mutual aid model, HHA members are able to empower each other to meet their own needs and create social change in the process. Another volunteer described the success and work of the organization: "The work is everyone. . . . The work is all of us."[40] In this way, the mutual aid framework of Health Action has destabilized the traditional hierarchies of patients and providers, of charity workers and beneficiaries. The mutual aid model flattens these hierarchies so that HHA members are brokering health care and accessing necessary medical supplies for themselves and each other.

Implications of the Philosophies of Care

The Third Net is an expansive yet ignored tier of health provision within the overall infrastructure of the US health care system, a tier composed of disparate organizations with varying structures, missions, and approaches to migrant health care. As the examination of these five migrant health organizations demonstrates, Third Net organizations largely share their reliance on volunteers, their provision of limited primary and preventative health care, and the negotiation of free or low-cost care within the mainstream health system for their patients. This analysis also reveals the wider limitations and resource constraints faced by all Third Net organizations working to provide migrant health services within a larger tiered and unequal health system. We argue that the philosophies of care adopted by each organization matter. These various approaches to migrant health care have larger implications for the way that Third Net organizations operate and their critiques of the health care infrastructure in the US (see table 1.2). First, philosophies of care impact the organizations' visibility and legibility. Those with more traditional philosophies of care are often the most visible of Third Net organizations and the most *intentionally* visible. This visibility is largely in their public-facing presence to potential funders, like government entities and foundations, but also to non-migrant individuals in the wider community. Social justice and mutual aid organizations may choose to maintain some invisibility to the wider public; they may not put a sign in front of the building or may not even have a building at all. Many Third Net organizations are established organizations with a public presence; others operate more informally and under the radar; and some have more clandestine operations out of people's homes or makeshift spaces. These varying levels of public visibility also have implications for the organizations' legibility as health organizations. In this case, more publicly visible organizations and those with more traditional philosophies of care are more legible to potential funders and to mainstream health entities and thus are able to access more financial resources, beyond individual donations, for their operations. In turn, organizational funding impacts the size of an organization, the number of patients it can accommodate, and the services it can provide.

Philosophies of care also influence what types of funding Third Net organizations are willing to pursue. For instance, of the organizations discussed in this chapter, those with traditional philosophies of care accessed grant funding from large foundations as well as from state and federal governments. The social justice and mutual aid organizations, on the other hand, did not access government or grant funding (although that is not necessarily the case with all social justice organizations). These Third Net organizations either were shut out from accessing grant funding due to not having 501(c)3 nonprofit status[41] or had made a conscious decision not to pursue funding that might require them to change their approach to care or compromise their ability to advocate for social change. As a result, the social justice and mutual aid organizations relied primarily, if not solely, on individual donations. This reliance on individual donations greatly constrains the amount of funding they are able to access as well as the investment of time and effort it takes to raise money for the organization. In turn, the organizations' funding structures also limit their size and the number of patients they can accommodate.

In addition to funding structures, the variability in visibility and legibility of Third Net organizations produces differences in their relationship to the infrastructure of the mainstream health system. Both traditional organizations maintain more formalized relationships with the overall health care system and safety net. For instance, Grace negotiated formal partnerships under the "Compassionate Care Partners" network of providers that deliver free health services to Grace's patients, while Centro has a selective referral system to the FQHC San Augustine's. By intentionally cultivating formal partnerships, these traditional Third Net organizations are fairly well integrated into the health infrastructure of the mainstream system. In contrast, these relationships among the social justice and mutual aid organizations in our study are less formalized, more ad hoc, and largely dependent on the existing social relationships and networks of the organizations' volunteers and members.

These variations in visibility, funding structures, and negotiations for health care access in the mainstream system are reflective of the fundamental differences in the mission and vision of the organizations. The traditional organizations in our study may privately have their own critiques of the US health and immigration systems, but these critiques do not shape the organization beyond the fact that they are providing health care to people who are otherwise unable to access it. The traditional free clinic, Centro, works to create a clinic space that approximates as closely as possible an FQHC, while Grace, as a traditional charity, works to provide free health care based on the principles of charity. As a result, their respective visions for the organization shape the care they provide and their interactions with their volunteers and patients. For social justice organizations in our study, both CommUnity Clinic of Phoenix and Justicia y Paz are providing free health care for their patients, like the traditional organizations, but they maintain a dual mission and vision that also includes a right to health care for all and the work to effect change around immigration and health in the US. For CommUnity and Justicia, they very much consider their health care provision and related work to be health care advocacy that challenges the failures of US health and immigration systems. Furthermore, CommUnity founders and volunteers are closely integrated with the migrant rights movement in Phoenix, who work to directly challenge anti-immigrant policy and rhetoric. For Houston Health Action as a mutual aid organization, the critique and social change demanded by the organization's mission and vision comes directly from the most marginalized and precarious uninsured, undocumented migrants with the most acute health conditions. In this way, their critique extends beyond immigration and health policy to also challenge issues that directly affect their members, including disability rights issues and even fare hikes for public transportation. Across Third Net organizations, then, there are a host of fundamental differences that shape not only individual organizational missions but also their larger vision for the society in which they should be operating.

Conclusion

Histories of free health care provision demonstrate different approaches to care for uninsured, indigent patients that have shaped the health safety net in the US. Philosophies of care in the Third Net draw from these various historical approaches in ways that shape organizations' missions, social relationships, larger critiques of inequity, and vision for social change. Through the examination of the work of five Third Net organizations and their various philosophies of care, this chapter has provided examples of the types and range of organizations within the Third Net. These various philosophies of care entail divergent and even contradictory missions and visions for migrant health care both locally and across the US.

The rest of the book will focus on further analysis of the three organizations in this chapter adopting social justice and mutual aid philosophies of care—Justicia y Paz, CommUnity Clinic of Phoenix, and Houston Health Action. Traditional free clinics like Centro de Salud and charities like Grace in Action are already the most visible and well-known Third Net organizations and have been analyzed in more detail in public and academic scholarship. Social justice and mutual aid Third Net organizations beg for further analysis in an age of increasing anti-immigrant policy and rhetoric and challenges to the health care infrastructure in the US. Social justice and mutual aid approaches to migrant health care enable a radical shift in the discourse and practice of free health care in the US and provide opportunities to re-envision social relationships by destabilizing power hierarchies between migrants and health practitioners.

Although the informality of the Third Net presents practitioners and migrants with notable challenges (e.g., steady funding and labor power), it also presents opportunities for everyone involved to advocate for a more just health care system. In practical terms, Third Net practitioners contend with more migrant health care demands than ever before. Philosophies of care within the Third Net do not simply involve facilitating access to care; they also can involve explicit challenges to anti-immigrant policies and rhetoric as well as to current hierarchies of health care access and provision in the US. The following chapters delve deeper into our ethnographic and interview data, giving shape to our theorization of the Third Net through the experiences and perspectives of the organizations' staff, volunteers, and to some extent patients. These chapters provide a clearer picture of the infrastructure of the Third Net and the ways that Third Net organizations provide care to their patients, negotiate patient access to limited health care services beyond the capacity of their organizations, and work to create more just immigration and health systems on a local level.

2

All Roads Lead to the Third Net

"We're not medical specialists, but to tell you the truth, we do a lot of medical work here," shares Margaret, director of Justicia y Paz (or Justicia for short), during a tour of the volunteer-run, community-based organization in Houston, Texas, that provides basic medical and non-medical provisions exclusively to low-income undocumented migrants. She directs us into a nondescript beige building that many would have never guessed was a clinic. "Doctors volunteer their time here once, twice, or three times a week, depending on their availability. Today is special, though, because we have our dentists. They usually only come once or twice a month. With so many people in need, we have to hold a raffle to see who gets to see the dentist."

We enter the clinic and it comes to life. Migrants converse in a couple of small waiting rooms immediately to the left of the entrance. Behind the check-in counter, a woman immediately notices our arrival and warmly greets us. Above her, a sign reads "We only and exclusively give care to undocumented people." Behind her, the check-in area extends back into a small room where four or five volunteers and dentists—indistinguishable from one another—juggle multiple tasks: filing away hundreds of patient information sheets; printing out copies of hand-drawn bus directions to other clinics, organizations, and legal aid agencies; and obtaining patients' weights, blood pressures, and temperatures.

Margaret guides us down a long hallway past two single-occupancy bathrooms, six patient rooms, and a medical closet filled with an assortment of equipment: gauze, bandages, alcohol wipes, blood pressure monitors, thermometers, and medical tape—all purchased with donated funds. We follow a scratching sound and poke our heads into one of the patient rooms. A man lays back on the chair with three people hovering over him ready to pull out his teeth. Tooth extraction, Margaret explains, is all dentists can do for migrants at Justicia. If every person in the waiting rooms has just one tooth pulled out today, the dentists will have extracted nearly 30 teeth.

The tour continues. We exit the clinic's rear entrance and walk across a long yard that stretches behind the clinic and a larger, two-story building where migrant women and young children temporarily reside, what Margaret calls the "women's house." A small playground and ten-foot-long clothesline sit on the grassy terrace, and further down, a tall wooden fence separates the yard from Justicia's sizable garden—an impressive lot of land cultivating long rows of fresh produce. Before entering the women's house, Margaret points to the back wall: "On the other side of the block is our 'men's house.'" The building is only one story but occupies a wider stretch of land than the clinic and women's house combined; it's almost half the other side of the block. The sounds of men's laughter and a Spanish music radio station pass through the wall.

We retreat into the women's house and follow Margaret through a large, tile-floored dining room with six long tables and more than 20 chairs.

"This is where we'll have lunch later," Margaret says. "The women and children sleep upstairs."

The dining room's walls are decorated with a mix of ESL lessons, an English-Spanish alphabet, and artwork depicting Catholic Worker Movement philosophy, which guides all of Justicia's activities. Next to the dining room are a small chapel, a playroom filled with toys and miniature brightly colored chairs, a walk-in pantry that stretches at least 20 feet, and a kitchen. The kitchen has two gas-powered ovens, four large sinks, two lockable freezer chests, and a sizable walk-in refrigerator filled with Spanish-labeled packages of boxed milk, cereal, spices, juice, bottled water, zip-lock bags, and foil. The top shelves are stacked with almost a hundred brown bags, each filled with a sandwich and the surprise of either an orange or an apple. These, we later learn, are reserved for the region's day laborers.

Margaret also shows us her office, the organization's library, and other storage rooms stacked with donations. The office feels tiny. It is filled with piles of organization newsletters and Harris Health financial assistance (i.e., Gold Card) applications, and in the corner of the room, a plastic container carries well over a hundred alphabetized prescriptions and over-the-counter drugs purchased on behalf of migrant patients.

Bulletin boards hang on the walls listing country codes and thumb-tacked photographs of smiling volunteers and migrant guests. The library is also small. It contains four dark brown bookshelves, offering readers ages five and younger an assortment of colorful, illustrative English-learning texts and several copies of books about the Catholic Worker Movement. Several other rooms serve as exclusive storage spaces for organization purchases and community donations: rice and beans, suitcases, cooking supplies, hygiene supplies, strollers, infant car seats, toys, and diapers.

Our tour concludes with one of the many meals shared each day at both the women's and men's houses, prepared with food either grown in the organization's garden or purchased from the Houston Food Bank. In both houses, the migrant guests are primarily responsible for preparing meals. A whiteboard in the women's house dining room displays the names of migrant guests responsible for cooking each meal and taking out the trash every day.

We finish our meal and thank Margaret for her time. As we leave Justicia, more migrants arrive.

* * *

To illustrate the centrality of the Third Net for those denied care and those eager to provide it, we center this chapter on the case of Justicia y Paz (Justicia), a Catholic Worker Movement–inspired[1] organization in Harris County (Houston, TX) that delivers broadly defined care (i.e., medical services, food, clothing, and temporary shelter) to hundreds of low-income undocumented migrants every year. The difference in scale between one of Houston's largest networks of health care providers—the Harris Health System (or simply Harris Health)[2]—and Justicia could not be starker. In fiscal year 2020, Harris Health's net revenue was approximately $1.71 billion;[3] Justicia's revenue was $0. Harris Health is made up of 18 community health centers, five school-based clinics, five same-day clinics, one dialysis center, one dental center, several mobile units, three multi-specialty clinics, and two full-service hospitals. In contrast, Justicia provides services across ten houses and small buildings. At any given moment, Harris Health employs thousands of professionally accredited physicians, medical social workers, interpreters, physical therapists, dentists, and clerical staff; at Justicia, there are usually no more than a handful of volunteer doctors and six full-time non-medical volunteers, many of whom have little to no professional medical training. Harris Health sits among a thousand acres of health care facilities, hotels, retail stores, and chain restaurants that make up Houston's colossal Medical District, or what *Forbes* contributor Scott Beyer calls "Houston's Medical Mini-City."[4] Justicia's primary operations, on the other hand, happen on one neighborhood block. Despite these distinctions, Justicia continues to survive, and we discuss how and why this is. Drawing on interviews and ethnographic observations with volunteers and migrants at Justicia, health practitioners, and Harris Health medical administrators, we argue that Third Net spaces like Justicia survive because they have entire infrastructures of their own. On the surface, Third Net spaces appear minuscule and delicate, but in actuality, they each have extensive infrastructures of support that keep them running and growing. The aim of this chapter is to illustrate how big the Third Net really is.

The Third Net's very existence is a consequence and critique of today's formal systems of care. The United States would not need a Third Net if private and safety net hospital systems sufficiently addressed the nation's vast health disparities. Houston's Harris Health System provides a telling case in point. By all accounts—size, revenue, and labor power— Harris Health easily stands as one of the most robust medical districts in the country. Yet, its coalition of safety net providers—those that provide care irrespective of patients' ability to pay[5]—struggle to maintain migrants as a health care focus. And this is precisely where Third Net spaces like Justicia come into play.

Amid an eroding welfare state, Justicia's efforts at promoting medical and social well-being for low-income undocumented migrants are both exhaustive and exhausting. Today, nearly 11.3 million undocumented migrants[6] are legally ineligible for health coverage, food stamps, employment services, and housing assistance, and as COVID-19 rages on, debates about their deservingness for such resources are intensifying. Consequently, the work of volunteers at Justicia is substantial, and the care they provide pertains to both medical and non-medical needs. Volunteers are responsible for mobilizing an extensive array of life-saving resources, navigating the slow, arduous frontlines of health care and legal bureaucracy, and moderating relationships and interactions. And, against pervasive dehumanizing, racist, and xenophobic discourses among politicians, the media, and some members of the public, they are responsible for justifying migrants' lives as inherently valuable, beautiful, complex, and important. When met with the common question asked of activists, community organizers, and academics—why is your work on migrant health care and social well-being important—most volunteers are taken aback, as if to respond, "why isn't it?"

Justicia is one of over 200 Catholic Worker Movement–inspired houses of hospitality[7] across the globe[8] and arguably one of Houston's best-known community-based organizations. It is situated in a rapidly developing urban neighborhood peppered with a mix of mid-rise condominiums, taquerias, hookah bars, churches, and storage facilities. Thanks to a unique lack of city-wide zoning laws, the organization's main buildings comfortably occupy an entire neighborhood block surrounded by booming businesses, late-night taquerias, and condo-building mania. Although Justicia serves one of the most multiply marginalized populations in the entire metropolitan region, it sits only blocks away from one of Houston's richest neighborhoods, a space where there is a Starbucks on three out of four corners of a single intersection. To urban developers, the organization is an eyesore, a missed opportunity for capital investment.[9] To migrants, it is a safe haven, a place to receive broadly defined "care" (medicine, food, shelter, etc.) while all other sources of medical and social support remain inaccessible.

Justicia teaches us two things about the Third Net. First, it illustrates how central the Third Net is to our existing health care and social infrastructure. What do social workers, community members, health physicians, law enforcement, and ICE officials all have in common? They all direct or bring low-income, uninsured, undocumented migrants directly to Justicia. Seven days a week, 24 hours a day, volunteers heed the calls of community members, police stations, hospitals, homeless shelters, and churches in search of migrant support, and every day they open the doors of Justicia to hundreds of undocumented men, women, and children each year from various regions of Latin America, the Horn of Africa, and the Philippines. Much like indigent citizens, low-income undocumented migrants do not simply "fall through the cracks" of a "broken" health care system, a phrase common among researchers and wider public alike.[10] "Cracks" are costly, and "broken" is a misnomer for a health care system firmly intact and intent on capital accumulation.[11] While federal law prohibits "patient dumping,"[12] Third Net spaces like Justicia operate as the de facto "dumping ground" for externalized migrant health care and resource provision. In taking on the arduous work of keeping migrants alive, Justicia simultaneously subsidizes ever-shrinking US welfare programs connected to health care, housing, and nutrition assistance. In combination with migrants' stories and experiences, volunteers' insights illustrate that migrants end up on the doorsteps of Justicia because the pipework of our health care and social infrastructure directs them there.[13]

Second, Justicia shows us how expansive the Third Net's own infrastructure is. All roads lead to Third Net spaces like Justicia, and from the Third Net, an entirely new internal infrastructure emerges. Volunteers from Justicia learn the blueprints of this internal infrastructure. In doing so, they provide a vantage point from which to understand institutional channels that *lead to* Justicia (i.e., an infrastructure of intentional patient dumping) and those that *extend from* Justicia (i.e., an infrastructure of support). Accordingly, we learn that the Third Net is not simply a linchpin of the formal health care system but also the heart of an extensive and robust network of individuals and institutional forces dedicated to mobilizing resources and meeting the needs of the people in ways that formal health care practitioners are unable to. While every Third Net space is different, Justicia illustrates just how far-reaching each organization's internal infrastructure can be. Justicia's internal infrastructure is massive, encompassing a network of organizations and allies across the Houston metro and religious institutions that literally span across the globe.

As highlighted in chapter 1, Third Net sites often operate with different philosophies of care but share a broader critique of the formal sector's inability to provide equitable care under a system designed to protect capitalist interests. From the vantage point of the Third Net, the formal and informal sector make up a single health care system that prioritizes profits and people differently (figure 2.1). Mapping Justicia onto this model, we see the centrality of the Third Net. From the top (i.e., the formal health care system), Justicia receives people in need of care. From the bottom (i.e., an extensive network of supporters), Justicia receives the resources needed to provide this care.

More recently, COVID illustrates how pervasive for-profit capitalist interests are in health care. Especially in moments of crisis, we expect

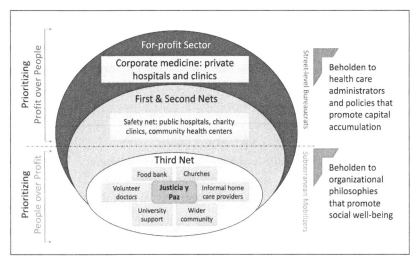

Figure 2.1. The US health care system: prioritizations of profits and people

social institutions to perform triage, or allocate resources to heal and support people, but in what sociologist Scott Schaffer calls the "necroethics of late capitalism," we are seeing the opposite: the allocation of people (predominantly people of color[14]) to heal and support resources—that is, "to essentially serve as profit fodder."[15] Today's health practitioners struggle to avoid this role.

Social scientists often regard practitioners (i.e., doctors, medical social workers, staff) across the for-profit sector and formal health care safety net (i.e., First and Second Nets) as "street-level bureaucrats" because they work *on the ground* (the "street" level, if you will) and implement health care administrators' and lawmakers' policies.[16] This makes practitioners in these formal settings beholden to two entities: 1) patients and 2) health care administrators. Within the context of increasingly privatized health care in the United States,[17] practitioners must not only ensure the well-being of patients but do so in coordination with the demands of higher-level administration and social policies designed to maximize production, minimize waste, and increase profit.[18] In short, practitioners are institutionally beholden to administrative directives and policies firmly focused on prioritizing *profits over people.*[19] This is not to suggest that practitioners in these settings are not compassionate, empathetic, or personally driven to directly help and heal people. Practitioners in these settings may have every intention of facilitating or providing patients' access to holistic, quality care, but neoliberalization of the entire welfare state embeds state-market rationality into most of their day-to-day operations,[20] making it difficult for them to avoid practices and bureaucratic protocols that prioritize capital accumulation over people's medical and social well-being. This is precisely how a health practitioner might sign off on an undocumented patient's medical deportation without knowing that they have done so.[21] However, Third Net practitioners are able to adopt a different aim.

Ethnographic and interview data illustrate that volunteers at Justicia—like other Third Net practitioners—fundamentally center on meeting the needs of the people; in short, they prioritize *people over profits*. Two things allow Third Net practitioners to do this. First, many Third Net practitioners who do, in fact, have medical training retain their employment within the formal First or Second nets. The formal sector—with its competitive salaries and larger operating budgets—gives health practitioners economic security, and this economic security allows health practitioners to volunteer their time with the Third Net for free. In short, the health care system's formal sector subsidizes the volunteer labor of medical providers in the Third Net.

Another reason Third Net practitioners are able to prioritize the needs of people is their general self-sufficiency and informal separation from the formal sectors of the health care system. The Third Net is distinct from but nevertheless connected to the other tiers of the formal health care system, which means it directly impacts the formal health care system but is not itself beholden to the same directives, rules, and policies as the formal health care system. In a sense, Third Net practitioners operate "below the surface," insulated from the neoliberal policies of profit maximization that govern formal health practitioners' day-to-day activities. In turn, we regard Third Net practitioners as *subterranean mobilizers*. Though very much "on the ground" and visible, subterranean mobilizers (i.e., Third Net practitioners) perform exhaustive labor that is informal, "underground," and in many ways, invisible. Put simply, they accomplish the very triage expected of formal sectors of society: they mobilize and distribute resources to protect and heal people. And this does not simply pertain to material resources. Third Net practitioners mobilize material goods (e.g., food, clothing, medical supplies), cultural capital (e.g., skillsets, ideas, beliefs),[22] and human capital (i.e., people, community organizations). Compelled by faith, justice, or some combination of the two, they have the drive to build and/or continue social movements. Of course, every Third Net space attempts to accomplish this differently, each with its own local contexts, experiences, and consequences. But as the case of Justicia exemplifies, every Third Net space operates with an internal infrastructure that resonates in some way with the aim of prioritizing the needs of people.

In the remainder of this chapter, we show how central an informal, community-funded Third Net organization like Justicia is to both those who need care and those eager to provide care. Justicia operates as an extension of the 1930s-inspired Catholic Worker Movement that continues to anticipate the state's inability to care for the poor and legislate compassion. Responding to this perceived inability, Justicia volunteers draw support from its internal infrastructure and directly address a range of low-income undocumented migrants' medical and social needs. Ultimately, the case of Justicia shows us how expansive the Third Net is. Though Justicia, like any Third Net space, contends with its own set of limitations, it exemplifies the contradictory frailty and strength of a Third Net space that literally keeps low-income undocumented migrants alive.

Justicia y Paz: Filling In Where the State Fails

Like other "houses of hospitality" designed to "serve the poor," Justicia is a nongovernmental organization spiritually and philosophically motivated by the Catholic Worker Movement. Dorothy Day and Peter Maurin co-founded the movement in Staten Island, New York, in 1933 during the Great Depression, a period when the state was clearly failing to meet the needs of the people. In their view, the state was too bureaucratic and impersonal to legislate dignity or compassion for one another.[23] In a critique of early capitalism's bourgeoning free-market philosophy, they argued that people only knew how to care about themselves, not each other. Serving as an inspiration to other prominent leaders of the mid-20th century, including anti-war priest Daniel Berrigan and Cesar Chavez, Day called for a spiritual revolution of people's hearts and minds where people could learn to see and care for one another as they would Christ. To facilitate this, Day, Maurin, and other followers of the movement since then (known as "Catholic Workers") created hundreds of "houses of hospitality" across the globe[24]—spaces where people could adhere to the seven corporal and spiritual works of mercy advocated in the New Testament's "Sermon on the Mount" (Matthew 25) and come to know Christ by knowing "the poor." "The poor" means something different to every house of hospitality and includes "disempowered populations" like the homeless or sex workers.[25] In 1980, Catholic Workers Margaret and Larry founded Justicia, a house of hospitality for low-income, undocumented migrants in Houston, Texas.

Like other houses of hospitality, Justicia practices the "works of mercy" by following four Catholic Worker Movement principles: pacifism, hospitality, voluntary poverty, and personalism.[26] While *pacifism* condemns violence, *hospitality* advocates compassion. In Day's view and Justicia's practice, social change is won by love, not war: this is the only way to get closer to God. This is what makes the work of the movement important to Catholic Workers (or volunteers). Echoing other volunteers at Justicia, Sylvia says, "The reason I came here in the first place was really because of my faith and because when you're serving these people, you're serving Christ." The "Sermon on the Mount" guides them to provide food to the hungry, shelter to the homeless, and company to the lonely; it's about providing care to those who need it.

Practicing hospitality effectively, however, requires adherence to the movement's principle of voluntary poverty. *Voluntary poverty* means rejecting the consumption and possession tenets of capitalism, sharing in the experiences of the poor, and relying exclusively on community support.[27] For Catholic Workers at Justicia, voluntary poverty means living with the migrants they serve, sharing community-donated resources (e.g., food and clothing), and attempting to limit consumption to those items grown from the organization's own community garden. When Justicia does partake in large-scale purchases, it tries to limit its purchases to local businesses, avoiding corporate giants like Walmart and Home Depot as often as possible.

Catholic Workers do not simply *provide for* the poor—doing so would be a form of "charity," which Day called a "word to choke over." In her view, the church advocated "plenty of charity [but] too little justice,"[28] and a true revolution of people's hearts and minds would require both. In a uniquely radical departure from faith-based organizations inspired by traditional Catholicism, Justicia attempts to combine charity and social justice; it synthesizes the compassionate orientation of conventional faith-based spaces with the anti-capitalist stance of secular social justice movements.[29] In order to synergize charity and social justice, Catholic Workers must give to *and* know the poor—either by living with them and experiencing their day-to-day material conditions or by bearing witness to these experiences. To facilitate the latter, Day and Maurin began a newsletter called *The Catholic Worker*, which continues to be published in various locales today.[30] Written by both Catholic Workers and house of hospitality guests, the newsletters generally share what it's like to be a Catholic Worker, recount the experiences of the poor, and articulate organizational needs (e.g., cooking supplies, toilet paper, clothes). Day and Maurin printed 2,500 copies of *The Catholic Worker* when they began the movement in the 1930s.[31] Today, Justicia mails approximately 42,000 bilingual (English-Spanish) newsletters four times a year to churches, Houston community members, and former volunteers throughout the United States and other select countries. Over the course of four decades, the organization has shared over 900 volunteer and migrant stories, not only detailing the consistent care work that Justicia accomplished over the years, but also advocating for systemic change of domestic and global policies that have catalyzed mass displacement. The resulting community support has been tremendous.

Margaret and Larry did not begin Justicia with a large government or community grant. They simply took inspiration from Dorothy Day, followed "the ways of the saints" and asked for the community's support. Margaret explains: "You pray and tell people what you're doing, and people donate. It just works." In both 2014 and 2015, this recipe of prayer and information dissemination resulted in well over $2 million in donated funds. Along with giving routine talks at local parishes,[32] Justicia's newsletters have drawn in donations in the form of money, food, and material goods like cookware, furniture, and clothes. This support comes from residents throughout the Houston region and parishes across the world, including the Vatican. Margaret says that although support for Justicia throughout the years has been "a little touch and go," she does not worry about the organization's future financial security: "From the beginning, there have been good-hearted people who have supported us. The main reason they support us is because there are no salaries." All the money that flows into Justicia goes "directly to the poor," and no one at Justicia makes a dime. Holland, a volunteer who facilitates the preparation and distribution of Justicia's newsletter and self-identifies as the organization's "unofficial accountant," estimates that Justicia spends over $4,000 a day—that's almost $1.5 million annually. This sounds like an impossible amount for a community-based, volunteer-run organization to spend until we consider everything Justicia accomplishes day in and day out. This includes but is not limited to things like paying for all of migrants' medications (any medications over $10), rent and utilities for all Justicia's houses, up to $800 a month for 125 migrants in need of long-term home care, and of course, food and other groceries. While many community-based organizations contend with insecure funding and apply for government support that can restrict or alter their goals and activities,[33] Justicia—like other houses of hospitality—avoids being beholden to external interests by relying solely on community support. This allows Justicia to practice the Catholic Worker Movement's final principle: personalism.

Personalism refers to taking personal responsibility and initiative in addressing needs, no matter how big or small. This can range from something as mundane as cleaning a bathroom to more urgent things like taking someone to the emergency room. In this regard, the philosophy of personalism broadens the conceptual scope of "care" to include medical well-being—alleviation of physical injuries, chronic diseases, and adverse mental/emotional health—*and* social welfare—strengthening of social networks, food and shelter, legal services, education, and employment assistance. Although Justicia operates as a registered nonprofit and maintains financial records for auditing purposes, it is not beholden to the conditions of state funds and does not need to justify its expenses to any financial institution. It can use the monetary support it receives from the community however it sees fit and address any need it recognizes. Margaret says, "We don't have rigid budget classifications. So if we see a need, we can respond to it." Sylvia, a volunteer, reiterates, "We can just choose how we're going to respond to everything—every need that comes up."

Sylvia provides an example, recalling an exchange between Hilda, a Salvadoran woman, and Margaret. Officials from the Salvadoran consulate informed Hilda that they could send passports to her children in El Salvador for $250, which would allow them into Mexico. When Hilda asked Margaret for this money, Margaret readily agreed, reached into a waist pack, and handed Hilda the money in cash:

> Margaret just decided to fork out $250 to make that possible, you know. She didn't have to apply to any treasury. She could just do that . . . She could just respond to that need, and now these passports are probably already in hand.

If Hilda had applied for economic assistance from a government office, she would have likely had to undergo a long application process, and depending on the office, this could have taken months. Instead, she simply asked Margaret for assistance, and Margaret provided it, a common occurrence at Justicia. Sylvia's presumption that the passports are "probably already in hand" is also indicative of the ease by which support is provided at Justicia. In some ways, this non-bureaucratic mode of hospitality is characterized as anarchism. Sociologist Harry Murray explains:

> Anarchism interacts with hospitality in several ways. First, it reinforces the notion of personal responsibility for the poor—one cannot leave one's brothers and sisters to the cold "mercy" of the state. Second, it reinforces the belief that bureaucratic forms of organization should be avoided at all costs in Houses of Hospitality. Third, it enhances the adversarial nature of interaction with state welfare agencies in advocating for the homeless.[34]

In Dorothy Day's view, the state interrupts people's capacities for knowing one another and meeting each other's needs. Having to jump through the hoops of state-sanctioned bureaucracy guarantees both impersonalism and a certain level of wasted energy. At Justicia, Hilda is not reduced to a number standing in the line of some heavily bureaucratized office. She is a person who wants to see her children, and Justicia makes this possible.

Poverty governance in the Third Net can look very different from formal institutions that provide social and medical resources. The informal and non-bureaucratic structure of Justicia not only allows for rapid response but also highlights a level of trust between migrants and Third

Net practitioners that may not necessarily exist in more formal settings. Hilda asked for monetary support, and on behalf of Justicia, Margaret provided it. Margaret did not question whether or not Hilda would actually use the money for the intended purposes. Theologist Mary Segers explains:[35] "If a person asks for funds, and the Catholic Worker has some (they depend almost entirely on contributions), that person receives the money, even if it is used to buy 'another pint.'" Catholic Workers do not question the authenticity of people's requests. In contrast, formal bureaucratic setups—whether related to health care or some other institution— assume people's untrustworthiness. For example, in order for welfare recipients in the US to receive support, they must show proof of their need and their deservingness through various bureaucratic hoops: income, checks, work requirements, drug tests, etc.

At Justicia, Hilda is a "migrant guest" who *asks* for money from an organization and larger social movement intent on meeting the needs of the poor. In any other formal setting, Hilda is a "customer" who *applies* for money from an institutionalized space that likely intends to make some sort of profit. In such formal settings, Hilda would need to provide information that allows the state to surveil Hilda and collect on debts. Catholic workers do not question whether or not migrants at Justicia have ulterior motivations. They simply observe or listen to a need and respond to it. Personalism is about trust.

Personalism means that anyone who comes to Justicia's doors is cared for—an anachronistic condition today. Comedian Sebastian Maniscalco jokes,[36] "[In the 1990s], your doorbell rang, that was a happy moment in your house . . . *Now* your doorbell rings, [it's like] get the hell down, somebody's outside!" While this attitude may be true of many people across the country, it is not true of Justicia or its Catholic Workers. Sylvia recalls a conversation with Meg, another volunteer, who referred to this dynamic as the "tyranny of the door":

> We were talking once about the door and just like how answering the door really monopolizes the day . . . Meg called it "the tyranny of the door." That is so [this place]. It will wait until you are in the furthest corner of the house and then the doorbell will ring, and you've got to come all the way back to the front and open the door, run into the eyes of whoever is out there and find out what they need.

Within the purview of the Catholic Worker Movement, if the doorbell rings, Christ is waiting to be cared for on the other side. Sylvia goes on to explain that she and Meg entertained the idea of installing a camera and intercom outside of Justicia to mitigate the in-person interaction, but they both realized that this would run contrary to the movement's principles:

> You have to open the door and you're face-to-face with the person . . . that is like the peak of personalism. It's that moment at the door: you physically go [to the door], open [it], and talk to the person [to] find out what they need. And there's also like a level of trust that's communicated right away because I'm a 20-year-old girl and I open the door and I'm like "who's there?"

In what Sylvia calls the "peak of personalism," Catholic Workers have a spiritual obligation to open Justicia's doors when the doorbell rings. Sylvia also emphasizes the trust involved in this interaction. Not only do Catholic Workers have to trust migrants *outside* of Justicia, but migrants have to trust Catholic Workers *inside* of Justicia. This trust is a key component of Third Net spaces. Health care coverage restrictions, public charge ambiguity, and visible state presence around private and public hospitals have contributed to documented and undocumented noncitizens' general distrust of the formal health care system, resulting in "chilling effects" whereby noncitizens avoid medical services altogether.[37] By contrast, Justicia is a space that migrants have come to trust. Whether they are in need of health care, food, or refuge, the principle of personalism means that Justicia will do everything it can to provide it.

Taken together, the Catholic Worker Movement's four principles help Third Net spaces like Justicia have a greater impact on migrants' lives than typical "shelters." Javier, a volunteer, explains:

> Shelter is a very neutral, almost cold kind of place where you sleep and get fed, and that's it. But Justicia is definitely not just a place that you come, eat, and sleep. This is a house of hospitality. People come here and they are taken care of. Volunteers can interact one-on-one [with migrants], which is something you do not think about when you hear the word "shelter."

Echoing a sentiment shared among other volunteers, Javier emphasizes personal interactions as a key feature of houses of hospitality. Made possible by adherence to the principles of personalism and voluntary poverty, these personal relations are what separate houses of hospitality like Justicia from shelters. Kelly, another volunteer, emphasizes, "If you're not focused on the personalism thing, you cannot do the corporal works [of mercy]. I mean, then it becomes charity." Justicia is not a space where migrants simply eat and sleep; it's a space where community is born. Migrants and Catholic Workers form friendships, share meals, attend weekly masses, celebrate quinceañeras, rejoice in the life of newborns, and honor the deaths of those who have passed. The combination of these experiences instills Catholic Workers and the movement's thousands of supporters with an intimate understanding of migrants' lives and invites social change on a personal, spiritual level. Echoing Dorothy Day, Margaret emphasizes that synthesizing charity and social justice means changing the way people live: "We can't separate [charity and social justice]. That's our philosophy . . . You have to change the system, but in order to change the system you also have to change hearts." Eradicating poverty requires a change in people's hearts and minds so that they see "the poor" as Christ-like figures deserving of care.

Critics of the Catholic Worker Movement often assert that houses of hospitality like Justicia address surface-level problems and do little to change the underlying social structure causing these problems in the first place, as is the movement's aim;[38] some volunteers call this the "band-aid critique." However, this critique reflects a false dichotomy between charity and social justice that Dorothy Day worked to clarify, and it fails to appreciate the very real impact Third Net spaces like Justicia have had on migrants' lives. For Henry, a doctor and former volunteer, understanding this impact simply requires imagining what life without Justicia would have been like for the thousands of migrants that have come to its doors:

> Think of the absence of the Catholic Worker over these past [several decades]. Think of it. If you can imagine the absence of it, think about the state that the immigrants would be in. Think about the opportunities lost, the minds lost, the kids that wouldn't have gone to college because of this . . . Or think of all the upper-class people who wouldn't otherwise

be donating and thinking about the poor and suffering immigrant and not having an opportunity to participate and alleviate that suffering. So, I think the impact is actually huge, and there's a lot of pieces to it and one of those pieces where citizens want to come in is the faith aspect of it. It is an act of faith.

Justicia has clothed, fed, housed, and provided basic medical care to thousands of migrants for over 40 years. It has helped adults navigate the legal battles of asylum cases and provided temporary lodging for women and their children trying to get out of abusive relationships. A school bus stops in front of Justicia every weekday to pick up young children eager to continue their education. Over a hundred migrant families frequent Justicia every month seeking assistance for rent and home care. Many migrants fill out applications for work and government assistance while living in Justicia. None of these experiences would have been possible in Justicia's absence, and at the very least, Justicia humanizes migrant suffering in ways that practitioners in formal settings may not be able to.

Henry explains: "Think of how many people come to the door and we really can't do anything for them but engage in that conversation and see them as a human being, [and knowing that this] has somehow helped their day." Physician professionalization[39] and legal medical bureaucracy in formal health care settings can restrict this level of personal engagement.[40] The informality of Third Net spaces like Justicia means practitioners/volunteers like Henry can care for migrants without regard for these restrictions:

> I'm so glad I have the free clinic as an outlet to serve people. Those are my happiest days—[the ones] in the clinic. I don't have to count beans. I don't have to worry about production and money-making or things like that. So the only reason it's a band-aid is because we're not all participating in it.

At Justicia, Henry feels liberated from the top-down profit-driven considerations of corporate medicine, and he believes this allows for a pathway toward systemic change. His suggestion that Justicia's practices are a band-aid solution only insofar as not everyone is participating in them resonates with other Catholic Workers' views and parallels

Dorothy Day's belief that revolution begins with people's hearts and minds. In Henry's words, "what good is the law" or structural change if people continue to see each other as less than human? As elaborated later in this chapter, the Catholic Worker philosophy that all migrants who come to Justicia must be seen as human beings, as part of the "deserving poor," has very real limits and consequences. But such a philosophy nevertheless inspires considerable support for Justicia, and this support translates into an array of medical and social provisions for migrants in need of care.

Although the religious, faith-based foundation of the Catholic Worker Movement may rouse wariness among some, its secular practicality and social justice implications are undeniable. Sociologists might make strange the fact that humanity is more readily recognized in the health care system's informal Third Net than its formal counterparts where people continue to be seen as (latently profitable) "patients" first, human beings second.

The Third Net: At the Center of Care-Seeking and Caregiving

"As Dorothy Day, the Catholic Worker Movement's co-founder, said: 'All we can do is put in a couple of loaves and fishes and hope that the lord transforms them,'" says Margaret, Justicia's director. "And so we put in a couple of loaves and fishes, and people like our loaves and fishes."

In the Bible,[41] Jesus transforms five loaves of bread and two fish into thousands and is able to feed a mass of people. By comparison, Justicia, a Third Net space, runs solely on community donations and feeds well over 10,000 people every year. Over 200 people—noncitizens and citizens alike—come to Justicia every Tuesday for its year-round weekly food distribution. Within the walls of Justicia, migrants and volunteers who live at Justicia share three meals a day all 365 days of the year. Taking into account that no one at Justicia makes a penny, this is an extraordinary feat, one that vividly illustrates the sheer scale of need at Justicia and the deficiency of the state. This is what the Third Net does: it operates as both description and critique—it both illustrates and condemns the failings of the state.

Life as a Catholic Worker of Justicia means constantly contending with the structural deficiencies of the state. Low-income, uninsured, undocumented migrants seek care at Justicia because of these structural deficiencies, and in turn, proponents of Catholic Worker philosophy try to provide care. Implementing the Catholic Worker Movement's philosophy of personalism, volunteers become familiar with the structural conditions that direct migrants to spaces like Justicia and mobilize across institutions to provide care that pertains to medical needs (e.g., basic primary care and long-term home care) and social needs (e.g., food, housing, and employment assistance). This is how Justicia turns five loaves of bread and two fishes into thousands.

"The Hospitals Call Us Every Day": Justicia y Paz Takes On Immigrant Health Care

Over a hundred city blocks away from Justicia sits a cluster of hospitals that outline Houston's skyline and make up one of the country's largest medical systems: the Harris Health System. Every single day, health administrators, physicians, lawyers, and social workers make decisions that directly impact the lives of millions of people, and at the end of the day, these decisions lead low-income undocumented migrants directly to Justicia.

"About 25% to 30% of the population of greater Harris County is uninsured or underinsured," shares Jerry, a Media Relations Specialist with Harris Health. He paints a picture for us about how dire the county's uninsured rate is. "That translates to roughly 1.2 to 1.5 million people. You can imagine that slice of the population. We only see 310,000 to 320,000 different individuals, so you can imagine that there's a lot more people out there [that don't receive care]. It doesn't mean that you always need health care, but when you do, where do you go?"

As is true for the rest of the country, most undocumented migrants and indigent citizens in Harris County rely on the health care safety net for care, and it's rapidly shrinking.[42] The logic of the Affordable Care Act (ACA) was that as more people gained health insurance, the need for the health care safety net would decrease over time, but this has not been true for Harris County. An official from the Harris Health System explains: "There's this sense like, okay, Affordable Care Act passed, now everyone's got insurance so you don't really need continued federal funding at that level. That's not true for us. For us, it's basically unchanged."

The need for health care safety net services has not changed in Harris County because the state of Texas decided to opt out of the ACA's provision for Medicaid expansion. The move was not a surprise for some like Travis, a Community Health Worker Trainer, who said, "What is considered a 'handout' in Texas is considered a health care 'entitlement' in California." Rather than expand Medicaid through the ACA, Texas decided to seek additional funding under the Social Security Act's 1115 Waiver,[43] which essentially allows local hospitals and hospital districts (e.g., Harris Health) to maintain decision-making power regarding what health care delivery looks like. Because the state did not expand Medicaid, over 770,000 Texans have ended up in a "coverage gap"[44] where they make too much to qualify for Medicaid but not enough to qualify for federal marketplace subsidies. The Kaiser Family Foundation estimates that 2.2 million US adults fall into the coverage gap, over a third of whom reside in Texas alone; if every state in the country expanded Medicaid in 2021, 4.3 million nonelderly adults would be eligible for coverage.[45] In Harris County, the health care safety net continues to be the only recourse for those in the coverage gap. Travis explained, "There's still a large amount of underinsured in this area. They don't quite qualify for ACA subsidy programs and can't quite pay for their care all on their own. So a lot of times, they're relying on these safety net programs."

In addition, the fact that Texas did not expand Medicaid has meant that safety net practitioners have had to provide uncompensated care for nearly the same percentage of uninsured patients (approximately 27% according to 2014 Census estimates) it had seen before the ACA, but with less federal funding. Harris County is home to the second-largest concentration of undocumented individuals in the nation, just behind Los Angeles County.[46] To stay afloat, health care safety providers have had to direct their focus more on "paying" (i.e., potentially Medicaid-eligible[47]) citizens and less on "gratuitous" (i.e., definitely Medicaid-ineligible) undocumented migrants.[48] Consequently, Justicia becomes one of the only avenues left for immigrant health care.

"The hospitals call us almost every day," says Margaret, Justicia's director. "We're relatively lucky in Houston. Other cities just call in an air ambulance and deport them." Here, Margaret references medical deportations[49]—where undocumented patients are forcibly repatriated to their home countries, often without their consent. In addition to hospitals, she receives calls from social workers, other community organizations, migrant families, and even law enforcement, all with the same request: can you provide care for undocumented migrants?

In alignment with Catholic Worker Movement philosophy, volunteers of the organization do not operate with a "someone else will help" mentality. During every conversation with Margaret, the organization's landline-based portable phone would ring, and she would answer it. It's telling that the organization does not have a voicemail system. Margaret remains vigilant and ready mentally and emotionally to respond to every call that comes to Justicia, seven days a week. The phone rings; Margaret answers it. Period. If the organization does not respond to these calls, Margaret rationalizes, who will? "In the mid-'90s, hospitals started calling about these very sick people who they wanted out of the ER. They took care of them and now it was time to go. And who's going to support them? We said, 'we don't do that.' But then we realized that nobody [else supports them] either." The paradox of Harris Health is that it is one of the largest medical systems in the country but calls on Third Net spaces like Justicia for migrant health care. "We started off with one or two people," Margaret explains. "They're still there. So you know, what can you say? They're paralyzed but they live."

The challenge is that Justicia is limited in its capacity to provide care for so many people. "The problem is that there's too many," Margaret says. "We can't take everybody because once we take people, we get them for years and years. And people ask us, 'well, how do you know you're going to have funds for next year?' We don't. And as Larry used to say, 'as long as they're alive and we're alive, we'll try.' But then that means that the risk is bigger and bigger."

The Emergency Medical Treatment and Active Labor Act of 1986 (EMTALA) forbids "patient dumping," but when low-income undocumented migrants need care, all roads lead to Justicia. According to Paul Stevenson, a doctor who has juggled work between Harris Health and Justicia since 1993, district hospitals like Ben Taub and Lyndon B. Johnson frequently send older patients and stroke victims directly to Justicia because they have nowhere else to go (many of them have been abandoned by their families) and because other spaces (e.g., the Salvation Army) are particularly discriminatory against Spanish speakers.

While migrants arrive at the doorsteps of Justicia every year for a variety of reasons, many come specifically for its clinic. Like all of Justicia's activities and services, the clinic runs solely on volunteer labor. Catholic Workers running patient intake and front-office tasks have little to no formal medical experience, and Harris Health–based doctors who volunteer their time at Justicia may or may not actually specialize in the types of medicine migrants need. Margaret explains:

> The Tuesday doctor is a family doctor, so he can see kids. The Thursday doctor is an oncologist at MD Anderson with a specialty in colon cancer, but he sees everybody [laughs]. So we're doing okay on that. And then Dr. Vazquez on Mondays has been coming forever. He's a chronic pain specialist. And then on Friday mornings, we have two doctors, a gastroenterologist and a neurosurgeon.

Doctors who volunteer their time at Justicia have an eclectic range of specialties. This also includes dentists who only perform tooth extractions and a pediatric ear, nose, and throat (ENT) specialist willing to see adults. "[The pediatric ENT] discovered that other specialists come in and do internal medicine, and so he decided to do it too," Margaret says. Only one general practitioner (i.e., family doctor) is mentioned. Volunteers hang up a monthly calendar outside the clinic showing what days of the week to expect certain doctors, but this information is not posted online. Moreover, doctors' specialties are not listed on the calendar itself; this information is conveyed only through word of mouth. Compared to a typical formal clinic setting staffed with individuals experienced in medical intake and more general health practitioners, Justicia's clinic runs with whatever it has. This is why a colon cancer specialist might see someone with debilitating migraines, or a gastroenterologist[50] might treat an individual for bug bites.

None of the doctors at Justicia have to be there, and this is significant for two reasons. First, the doctors who volunteer their time at Justicia are motivated to help people, not make "a buck." Although they receive no compensation for their services and likely work with fewer forms of support (trained staff, medical equipment) than they may be used to, they keep coming back. As indicated above, Henry, a doctor and former volunteer, feels liberated by the Justicia clinic: "I don't have to count beans. I don't have to worry about production and money-making or things like that." Like other doctors, Henry recognizes the clinic at Justicia as a space where he can prioritize the needs of patients without being buried under stacks of paperwork. Neither Henry nor his patients have to worry about medical bureaucracy in order to provide or receive care, respectively. In the formal health care system, migrants without an ID might be denied care and face a cascade of consequences.[51] At Justicia, they don't need an ID or a page of documentation to receive care. The second reason doctors' voluntary presence at Justicia is significant is that they play a key part of the Third Net's internal infrastructure of support. Volunteer doctors are the very reason a Third Net space like Justicia is able to provide low-income undocumented migrants basic health care provisions, ranging from medical gauze and skin ointments to wheelchairs and life-saving medications.

Migrants' stories draw many volunteer doctors to Justicia. Most learn about the organization through word of mouth, the organization's newsletter,[52] or church services, all of which provide testament to migrants' experiences and act as a mobilizing force for support. "The archdiocese here allows us to give talks in the parishes, and so we have done this for years," shares Margaret. "When we give those talks, we mention the clinic. We don't get many dentist takers, but in the last couple of years, two doctors have come from those talks. One comes every Thursday afternoon, and now one's coming every Tuesday afternoon." When Margaret talks to members of the community, she shares stories about Justicia and its "migrant guests." Like the newsletters, her talks inform members of the community about the violence and hardships migrants have endured while crossing the border and living in Houston. These talks also convey what it means to be a Catholic Worker and serve Christ. Within the broader scope of the Catholic Worker Movement, the purpose of sharing migrants' experiences is to elicit a change in people's hearts and minds—to incite what movement co-founder Dorothy Day called a spiritual revolution where people treat each other with the same respect and love they would offer to Christ.[53] On a practical level, migrants' stories elicit support for the organization, be it money, material, or voluntary labor.

Justicia's clinic is itself a patchwork system that relies on donated medical supplies and volunteer doctors who, despite their best efforts, are unable to meet all the patients' needs. Kiara, a 20-year-old volunteer who regularly helps out at the clinic, observes the challenges doctors face:

> One time, there were almost 40 people at the clinic and only one doctor. More people were still coming, but we couldn't see them because we had to be fair to the doctor. We couldn't make him stand on his feet for like five hours to see everyone . . . And some doctors have to work like 80 or more hours a week. You would want them well-rested before putting patients' lives in their hands.

In most cases, doctors volunteer their time at Justicia at 6:00 a.m., see patients until 7:30 a.m., and then rush off to one of Houston's hospitals or clinics to begin day-long shifts. Care is provided on a "first come, first served" basis, and doctors agree to different patient loads. Some will see up to 25 people; others will take no more than 10. Accordingly, volunteers take down the names of migrants who show up to the clinic first—sometimes hours in advance—and create a list of patients being seen on a given day. Getting to the clinic is not easy for many undocumented migrants, and many of them rely on peers or public transportation. And after taking the time to travel several miles to Justicia's clinic, they may find it already full, or, as several volunteers share, the doctor may not even show up. Justicia's clinic does what it can, but the need is simply too great.

"If we could have someone at the clinic all the time, it would help the process," says Carolina, a 24-year-old woman who has volunteered at the clinic for nearly six years. "Just a full-time clinic would be great." Despite providing invaluable care for undocumented migrants in the Houston region, the clinic lacks the staff and resources to operate on a full-time basis. This leaves volunteers with two options: 1) help migrants care for themselves, eventually resulting in informal home care, or 2) help migrants get a "Gold Card," which provides limited access to the formal health care safety net on a temporary basis.

Informal Home Care

When it comes to chronic illnesses that require sustained attention, self-care and informal home care are generally all Justicia can offer, and they go hand in hand. "We have to teach people to take care of themselves," stresses Dr. Silva, a retired endocrinologist. He brainstorms with Margaret, Justicia's director. "People could consider a do-it-yourself option for dialysis."

"We should do that!" Margaret responds excitedly. "Do you know of people who would volunteer to go to people's homes and teach them how to do that?"

"Yes, let's discuss it. I'm sure we can do it."

These types of exchanges are common at Justicia. Like other doctors who volunteer at the organization, Dr. Silva recognizes the limits of care there and considers ways to enable migrants and their families to care for themselves in their own homes. This becomes particularly relevant when needs for long-term care emerge.

Informal home care is often the solution to migrants' long-term care needs. Whether it's because of the development of new conditions (e.g., strokes or heart attacks) or conditions that have exacerbated over time (e.g., diabetes, kidney failure, Alzheimer's, dementia), health practitioners, medical social workers, and migrant families all turn to Justicia for long-term care—about 125 people at the time of our study. Whereas citizens can generally draw on Medicare and Medicaid assistance to subsidize the costs of this care, undocumented migrants remain ineligible for such coverage, making institutionalized settings like nursing homes financially impossible. In 2020, the estimated national average per person cost for private nursing home care was almost $9,000 per month; in Texas, this cost was nearly $7,000 per month.[54] Comparatively, Justicia can only afford to pay each informal care home up to $800 per month for long-term care. With nursing home care out of the question, informal home care is the only type of long-term care left for many migrants. In many cases, however, the arrangements of these spaces are dire.[55] "Many people just gut their homes and fill them with beds," shares Dr. Stevenson. Over time, Justicia has identified particular homes where migrants are well cared for, but there are not many. "These are not good places. This is truly Dickensian. This is health care for the slave class."

Dr. Stevenson's characterization of informal home care as "health care for the slave class" illustrates two things. First, it emphasizes the poor quality of these spaces. Unlike formal home care settings where caregivers are medically accredited via state programs, informal home care operates with the labor of private residents and/or migrant families who likely have no medical training. Private residents often do not speak a word of Spanish, and given the informal structure of these spaces, migrants are not afforded the same legal protections as in formal settings. As a result, migrants routinely find themselves isolated in substandard conditions for long periods of time.[56] Second, in referring to informal home care as "health care for the slave class," Dr. Stevenson recognizes an important pattern in terms of who relies on such care. Many who depend on informal home care are part of a larger disenfranchised population of people without any legal or social recourse for long-term care. In this context, "slave class" refers specifically to undocumented migrants, but across different spaces and varying points in time, such a characterization can expand to include other multiply marginalized populations who find themselves locked out of the health care system.

Ultimately, the main beneficiary of these informal care homes is the formal health care system itself. Long-term care is expensive, and informal home care serves as a cheaper alternative. Rather than absorb the economic and labor costs of providing long-term care to low-income undocumented migrants, the formal health care system externalizes these costs to informal care homes.[57] Thus, the First and Second Nets of the health care system direct migrants to Justicia for long-term care, not just for the sake of migrants' well-being, but also for the sake of protecting the formal health care system's profits. And, while private hospitals fill their beds with patients and make millions every year,[58] households that provide informal home care to migrants make, at best, just under $10,000 annually regardless of how many migrants are cared for. Accordingly, those who provide informal home care act as an important extension of the Third Net. Despite the precarity of some informal care homes, caregivers in these settings provide long-term care that is otherwise virtually nonexistent for low-income undocumented migrants. In some ways, this echoes the sentiment Margaret shares above about migrants' conditions at Justicia: "they're paralyzed but they live." Informal home care is the best the Third Net can manufacture out of a health care system intent on protecting capital interests. In short, by exploiting the Third Net's prioritization of people over profits, the formal sectors of the health care system can continue focusing on profits over people.

The Gold Card

Given Justicia's limited clinical resources, Catholic Workers do every-thing they can to enroll low-income undocumented migrants in Harris Health's annually renewable financial assistance plan: the Gold Card.[59] As Margaret explains, doing so helps the organization maximize the number of migrants it can see in its own clinic: "We really do try to get them a Gold Card to move them into the system so that we could make space for others coming in." The Justicia clinic only sees undocumented migrants without other forms of insurance; if they have a Gold Card, they're redirected to clinics within Harris Health.

Since December 2000, the purpose of the Gold Card has been to pro-vide Harris County residents a sliding-scale discount for medical ser-vices within the Harris Health System.[60] According to Elisa, a Harris Health Community Health Training Specialist, the program sets Hous-ton apart from other Texas cities:

> I think Houston is unique in the sense that we have Harris Health, and with Harris Health, you don't necessarily have to have insurance. You can qualify for their assistance plan [the Gold Card]. So I think it's easier for people not covered by Medicaid or Medicare to use Harris Health because you don't have to be paying a premium. You just pay for services you receive.

Harris Health is a game changer for indigent populations, particularly those in the coverage gap. Gold Card patients do not have to pay a pre-mium for services, and depending on their income, other health care expenses can be drastically reduced.

Applications for the Gold Card "keep coming," shares Jim, an Eligibil-ity Specialist with Harris Health. He says the office can expect to process 42,000 to 44,000 financial assistance applications every month, 80% of which are renewals. The Harris Health System's *Policy and Regulations Manual*[61] characterizes the Gold Card as a "final option" and tempo-rary alternative to health insurance.[62] Recipients are expected to even-tually apply for and transition into Medicaid, Temporary Assistance for Needy Families (TANF), and/or Supplemental Security Income (SSI) at some point, but undocumented migrants are ineligible for these federal programs. Therefore, the Gold Card program is the only de facto form of health coverage undocumented migrants in Harris County are eligible for. The Gold Card covers up to 100% of expenses incurred within the Harris Health System, depending on the plan individuals qualify for.[63] This includes mental health services and prescription medications. Because undocumented migrants at Justicia have no source of steady income, they are eligible for the Gold Card's "Plan 0," relieving them of liability for any medical expenses.

To qualify for the Gold Card, however, individuals need three proofs: 1) income, 2) residency, and 3) identity. For most migrants, these proofs pose significant challenges.[64] In terms of income, undocumented migrants routinely engage in informal types of labor where they do not receive official pay stubs, tax forms, or state records reflecting their annual income. This allows employers to claim that they did not know they hired undocumented migrants, which became illegal with the 1986 Immigration Reform and Control Act. "Employers don't sign these forms because they're afraid the government will get them for hiring an undocumented person," Margaret shares. Another challenge is proof of residency. Many migrants do not have apartment leases, utility bills, school records, or other official documents with their address and names. This was the case for Julio, a diabetic Mexican who returned to Justicia solely for Gold Card support. Julio left the organization after finding housing with some friends but then returned almost immediately because his name was not on the apartment lease, and he needed proof of residency for a Gold Card. Without it, he was incurring nearly $200 worth of medical costs for every clinic visit he made. Margaret allowed Julio to return and fill out a "Harris Health System Agency Letter"[65] verifying his residency at Justicia. Because Justicia serves only low-income individuals and is situated in Harris County, the "agency letter" serves as proof of both income and residency. Margaret says,

> I don't know what we would do without our own clinics and . . . connections with the hospitals, which are very supportive in the sense that if we sign forms for people that live here, then [Harris Health will accept that as] proof of residency and income. . . . All they need is a good ID, which is problematic because some people don't have it.

Though Justicia can assist in proof of income and residency, proof of identity becomes an entirely different obstacle. State-issued driver's licenses, employee badges, student IDs, US immigration documents, passports, and foreign consulate ID cards serve as valid proofs of identification needed for a Gold Card, so long as they have individuals' pictures on them. If someone does not have one of these, they need any two of the following: birth certificate, marriage license, hospital records, adoption papers, current Harris County voter card, check stubs, Social Security card, and Medicaid/Medicare card.[66] For migrants who have lost or had their legal documents stolen and have no connections back home to obtain new documentation (via local consulates or embassies), proof of identity poses a significant challenge, and for many, it can become a death sentence.[67]

The Gold Card provides a lifeline for undocumented migrants. Without it, migrants incur exorbitant costs or risk forgoing care altogether. For example, the Gold Card saved Efren, a 60-year-old undocumented Mexican man, thousands of dollars after an open-heart surgery. He paid $5 and $15 for medicines that would have cost him $1000 and $3000, respectively, without a Gold Card. Margaret shares another example about Martin, a 60-year-old migrant man who had gone without insulin for nearly a year because his Gold Card expired: "Martin really wants to work as a roofer. I hope he doesn't, of course, because he doesn't have feeling in his hands and feet already." For migrants who have lost toes or feet because of diabetes, Justicia has numerous crutches, canes, and wheelchairs on hand, all of which have been donated to or directly purchased by the organization. The sheer quantity of these donations illustrates Justicia's understanding that it is not a matter of *if* migrants will need this support, but *when*.

This expectation of need sharply contrasts with formal sectors of the US health care system. The system's lack of ventilators when COVID-19 hit the country in 2020 provides a case in point.[68] It only took weeks for the United States to run out of ventilators, illustrating that the system was never prepared for a crisis of this scale. Sociologist George Ritzer[69] explains that the US health care system routinely adopts a "just in time" capitalist approach to resource provision, which means that it orders necessary resources and *responds* to crises *after* they have begun. This is a cheaper option in the short term than a "just in case" precautionary approach where hospitals and clinics order necessary resources and *prepare* for crises *before* they have begun. Like other Third Net spaces, Justicia adopts a "just in case" approach. It has to. Catholic Worker Movement philosophy prescribes distrust of the state's ability to meet the needs of the people, and Justicia plans accordingly. Thus, we see a different type of logistical work between the formal health care system and the Third Net: logistical work in the former involves maximizing efficiency and economic returns; logistical work in the latter involves mobilizing resources and support to optimize care.

Justicia's efforts to facilitate migrants' Gold Card enrollment are significant for two reasons. First, Third Net spaces like Justicia are the only spaces explicitly focused on immigrant health care. One of Harris Health's primary initiatives is Medicaid enrollment—that is, attempting to enroll as many people into Medicaid as possible in order to 1) expand patient coverage and 2) broaden the pool of "paying" patients to keep the safety net funded and afloat. One coalition responsible for this initiative is Enroll Gulf Coast, made up of eight partner organizations[70] that each focus on a different population in Houston (e.g., LGBTQ, Latinx, Asian and Asian American). During one Enroll Gulf Coast meeting, representatives from each of the eight organizations took turns sharing how many new people they had enrolled in Medicaid and plans for future enrollment. After the groups finished presenting, we asked a few of the coalition's members about the health care plan for undocumented migrants. As if we had just asked about a deceased relative, their facial expressions sank immediately. They looked at one another and then shook their heads: "we don't know." Health care for undocumented migrants is not on their radar. This was a pattern. When asked about immigrant health care, most Harris Health administrators and practitioners responded with silence. Others, however, emphasized the importance of other non-governmental spaces that provide care—that is, the Third Net.

"Most of the places where uninsured, undocumented immigrants go for care are non-profits that are funded through their own funding mechanisms and focus on specific populations," explains Travis, a Community Health Worker for Harris Health. The type of space he describes is precisely the Third Net. He shares that many migrants from Vietnam and the Middle East rely on Asian outreach and Muslim community centers in different parts of the city. Meanwhile, word-of-mouth advice and social worker direction leads many migrants from regions of Latin America directly to the front doors of Justicia. Thus, Justicia is just one of several non-governmental community-based organizations focused on the needs of migrants in Houston, and Harris Health knows it. The reason immigrant health care can be off Harris Health's radar is because Harris Health knows it can rely on the Third Net to pick up this work, and there are no consequences for this neglect. Immigration and health care law legally inhibits migrants from accessing primary-level care in the formal sector of the health system, ultimately forcing migrants *and* health practitioners to rely on emergency rooms[71] and the Third Net. Moreover, in clear illustration of what migration and health scholars call "medical legal violence,"[72] reliance on the Third Net is *normalized*, understood among Harris Health practitioners as *the* protocol for addressing migrant health. Moreover, Harris Health understands that Third Net spaces like Justicia can facilitate migrants' access back into the formal health care safety net via programs like the Gold Card.

Correspondingly, the second reason Justicia's Gold Card enrollment efforts are significant is that the Gold Card serves as a local loophole to federal restrictions in health coverage. As discussed in the introduction, one of the chief reasons the Affordable Care Act was able to pass was that it explicitly kept undocumented migrants ineligible for Medicaid and state exchange participation. The federalist nature of the US legal system[73] allows local governments to establish legal rules and conditions that do not neatly line up with federal law.[74] Medical districts *can* establish programs to allow low-income undocumented migrants access to forms of health insurance without calling it insurance. Thus, Harris Health's Gold Card program serves as an important, albeit temporary, backdoor to health coverage for low-income undocumented migrants in Harris County, and again, both Justicia and Harris Health know it.

The Gold Card is like a legal underground pipeline that keeps the formal health care safety net (Harris Health) and informal Third Net (Justicia) connected. Harris Health uses the Gold Card to create a set of conditions that allow noncitizens to obtain some form of health coverage. In turn, Justicia does everything it can to help migrants fulfill these conditions. This setup illustrates a collaborative relationship between the formal health care system and the Third Net: Harris Health calls on Justicia every day to care for noncitizens, and conversely, Justicia directs noncitizens to Harris Health after Gold Card conditions are met. Though distinct, the formal health care safety net (i.e., Harris Health) and the informal Third Net (i.e., Justicia) can use the Gold Card collaboratively to contest migrants' exclusion from the health care system. Although practitioners from Harris Health are verbally soft-spoken about provisions for undocumented migrants, Harris Health's website includes information explicitly tailored toward noncitizens.[75] With the Gold Card, Harris Health creates a set of conditions that can make noncitizens eligible for health care coverage, but it's up to Third Net spaces like Justicia to help migrants fulfill these conditions. In turn, Justicia volunteers work with migrants to fill out Gold Card applications. Sometimes, this involves gently emphasizing certain eligibility criteria. Margaret explains: "Fortunately, the Gold Card does not depend on legal status. Well, it does in the sense that if you ever had a visa . . . they won't let you have a Gold Card." When asked why having a visa might matter to the hospital district, Margaret responded, "The county supervisors said, through the politicians, that if we allowed people with tourist visas or those who overstayed their visas to have a Gold Card, the whole country of Mexico would come here. [*scoffs*] Please. I mean they have doctors in Mexico." Here, Margaret characterizes the hospital district's policy around visas and Gold Card applications as folly and unnecessary. However, she also recognizes the legal trouble Justicia could get into if they directly instructed migrants to withhold information. To reconcile these sentiments, she and other volunteers do not explicitly tell migrants to omit visa information on their Gold Card applications; they simply highlight the fact that having a visa disqualifies them from getting a Gold Card and then leave it up to migrants to fill out the applications however they decide.

The relationship between Justicia and Harris Health highlights the importance of local context in Third Net effectiveness. Justicia could not reintegrate migrants into the formal health care system without Harris Health's Gold Card program, and nothing legally compels Harris Health to make the Gold Card accessible to migrants. In other Texas locales, migrants have fewer options. Dr. Stevenson shares, "You're shit out of luck in Dallas, and Galveston has a coldness about it [where] doctors want to kick migrants' asses back to Mexico." Local context matters. As a major migrant hub, a sanctuary city, and one of the most ethnically diverse metropolitan regions in the country,[76] Houston can be understood as a predominately pro-migrant city, which cannot be said of other locales. This is to say that one of the central reasons Harris Health practitioners can be part of the Third Net's infrastructure is that the local politics of the city permits it.

"We Don't Usually Bother Churches": Caring for Migrants' Social Needs

Several migrants at Justicia recall instances when law enforcement and Immigration and Customs Enforcement (ICE) agents came to the organization not to pick people up, but rather, to drop people off. When Margaret, Justicia's Director, was asked why she believes this occurs, she responded that it's "probably because Justicia frames its operations in terms of the works of mercy [and] takes homeless and sick people off the streets." Referencing her late husband, Larry, she elaborates:

> We're not transporting people or anything like that. In the late '80s, Larry was on a panel of four people talking about immigration, and one of the panelists was the district director of immigration. During the session, someone from the audience [pointed at Larry and] asked, "why don't you arrest him?" And then the man from immigration kind of stuttered and said "well, we usually don't bother churches."

If one were to search for a list of "churches" in Houston, Justicia would not come up. Yet, its Catholic Workers credentials emit a religious aura of protective "sanctuary"[77] so compelling that even state officials do not feel they can "bother" it.

This philosophy of care is powerful. Every newsletter the organization sends out details the experiences of migrants,[78] shares the efforts of Catholic Workers in meeting migrants' needs, and, most importantly, invites the wider public to participate in the Catholic Worker Movement— that is, to adopt Catholic Worker philosophy to serve Christ through serving the poor, which in the context of Justicia means low-income undocumented migrants. Only once, during Justicia's Christmas issue of the newsletter, does the organization explicitly ask for economic support, and the result is a stream of over a thousand personally written letters, each expressing words of support and filled with cash or checks ranging from 10 dollars to thousands of dollars. For much of the wider public, this is how they get to participate in the Catholic Worker Movement, and in turn, this is how they act as a part of Justicia's internal infrastructure.

Margaret dedicates much of her time to responding to donation letters, a task she used to do with Larry before he passed away. While sometimes calling on the help of other volunteers at Justicia, Margaret responds to literally hundreds of donation letters each day with personalized, handwritten thank-you notes. These notes are made out to social workers, doctors, lawyers, journalists, researchers, former volunteers, clergy members from all around the world, and of course other residents in Houston. While other formal nonprofit and nongovernmental organizations may reprint the same thank-you note to their supporters, Margaret recognizes the importance of personal correspondence that conveys sincerity and authenticity. After all, the money that comes with these donation letters acts as the organization's lifeblood. An important distinction between the Third Net and its formal counterparts is that the Third Net can conceptualize "care" in broad ways. Of course, this can look slightly different in each Third Net space, but at Justicia, "care" refers to both medical *and* social needs. In this way, the Third Net has the capacity to provide a wider range of care than its formal counterparts, which center exclusively on medical provisions. Thus, Justicia's internal infrastructure is made up of people and institutional forces that contribute not only to migrants' medical needs but also to their associated social needs, including the need for food.

"Anyone who is poor can come for food," says Kelly, a volunteer. Justicia holds a food distribution at the women's house every Tuesday morning. Although the distribution begins at 6 a.m., the lines begin forming as early as 4:30 a.m. and generally stretch over a hundred feet long. Once inside, those who have come for food encounter an assembly line of volunteers, migrant guests who live at the men's house, and retirees, who each hand out a different food item. Every week comes with its own assortment of produce: bags of potatoes, cabbage, onions, oranges, and apples. Other items include rice, beans, boxed milk, green beans, instant mac and cheese, and canned corn. The distribution generally ends by around 8 a.m., and by then, it would be a miracle if any food remained.

Although unsure of the exact figures, Patrick, a retired man who usually runs the distributions, says that Justicia uses donated funds to buy approximately $7,000 worth of food from the local food bank every week.[79] Patrick explains that grocery stores around town usually give outdated food to the food bank, and in turn, Justicia purchases it for a reduced price. So essentially, people who come to the food distributions get whatever is left behind in larger grocery store chains like Whole Foods, Walmart, or Krogers.

"Sometimes the food we get is on the edge of being spoiled," Patrick says. "That's just an issue we have to take up with the food bank. Fortunately, though, we have Noland." Noland is an attorney who sits on the board of the food bank. If Justicia experiences any problems with the food they receive, Noland is quick to set things straight. "It's nice to have Noland because he donates a lot of time and effort. For example, every Thanksgiving he donates like 1,200 frozen turkeys to Justicia. We just have to pick them up."[80]

The food bank plays an enormous role in Justicia's internal infrastructure. Over 200 people come to Justicia's weekly food distribution, and on certain holidays like Thanksgiving, this number nearly triples. In the same way that people rely on underground pipes to pump clean accessible water every day, many in Houston rely on the invisible infrastructural link between Justicia and the food bank.

Another of Justicia's main activities is distributing brown-bagged lunches to day laborers in the region every day. With almost a hundred day laborers in the region, preparing these lunches takes a lot of time and labor, and Justicia relies on local parishes. "There's a lot of people out there wanting to help the poor, but they don't know how, so they do it through Justicia," explains Margaret. "You know, one of the churches nearby brings us sandwiches every week. They have 150 people involved in making those sandwiches."

Every week, Sandy, a woman from a local church, drives up to the front of Justicia in her compact sedan, opens her trunk, and carries in several boxes full of brown-bagged lunches. Volunteers then store them on a shelf in Justicia's walk-in freezer among well over a hundred other bagged sandwiches from previous weeks. Each sandwich is simple—just a couple of pieces of bread with cheese, various lunch meats, and a mayo spread—but reflects the personal work of someone devoted to feeding the hungry. The volunteers use their own funds to purchase the food and bags and devote substantial time to preparing them. The work parishioners put into preparing these sandwiches is almost invisible, appearing simple or mundane to most people, but it is important. On the occasional days when Justicia runs out of sandwiches, day laborers simply don't eat.

In addition to food, churches also provide Justicia with an invaluable resource: volunteers. Many people who come to live and volunteer at Justicia learn about the organization through their own congregations or universities. Cynthia recalls: "I was still trying to figure out jobs and stuff and then Larry and Margaret came to speak at my church. I was like, 'this is divine providence.' It was like a sign that I couldn't ignore, so I came here." For Sister Consuelo, a nun based out of San Antonio's Sister of the Sacred Heart congregation, Justicia was the best site for her to continue her congregation's objective of serving the poor: "The head of my congregation found Justicia for me. It aligns with our congregation's objective to go to the poorest of the poor. That's our mission. That's why I'm here." Amanda found Justicia through her professor's mother-in-law:

I ended up finding Justicia through a school connection . . . My professor knew that I was very Catholic and said, "you should call my mother-in-law. She's also super Catholic. You'd love her." So I called her and chit-chatted a bit, and then she said, "if you're looking for a place to serve, you should come live with me in Houston. I'm friends with this couple, Larry and Margaret, and they run Justicia." Then I found out it was a Catholic Worker house and was like, "perfect!"

Like Cynthia, Sister Consuelo, and Amanda, many volunteers initially learn about Justicia through personal networks formed in churches and universities, and all of them are drawn to the Catholic Worker Movement philosophy of service to the poor. Whether from Houston, other Texas cities like San Antonio, or faraway locales like New York, people who make the trek to volunteer at Justicia do so because the organization resonates with a consistent desire to meet human needs in a direct impactful way. By offering Third Net spaces like Justicia a relatively steady stream of volunteers, churches and universities act as an important part of Justicia's internal infrastructure.

The Limits of Care at Justicia

"There are a million things to do," says Sylvia. "But there is a point where you have to be like, 'okay. I'm not all powerful here. I can only do so much.'" Justicia has its limits. All Third Net spaces do. Despite the scale and scope of the Third Net, it cannot possibly do everything. Gaps in the Third Net are both structural (e.g., limited resources and labor power) and ideological (e.g., organizational philosophies). At Justicia, three limitations exist: 1) volunteers without medical training routinely have to serve as medical professionals, 2) migrants remain at the bottom of the organization hierarchy, and 3) the organization's entire internal infrastructure relies on the image of "the suffering migrant."

Non-medical Volunteers Who Do Medical Work

As shared at the beginning of this chapter, Director Margaret aptly summarizes the scope of Justicia: "We're not medical specialists, but to tell you the truth, we do a lot of medical work here." This statement captures determination and limitation. Volunteers do everything they can for low-income undocumented migrants who come to Justicia, but given their lack of medical training and experience, they can only do so much. Within the organization's clinic, volunteers' jobs are pretty straightforward: assist in patient intake, maintain patient records, and provide whatever support they can to doctors volunteering at the organization. Outside of the clinic, however, volunteers' labor is less defined and more situational.

For example, Frank, a volunteer in his mid-20s, lives at the men's house and acts as the de facto "medicine man." Sometimes, instead of asking for Frank by name, the men will ask for "el doctor," despite the fact that Frank has neither a medical degree nor a single day of formal medical education. Unlike migrants, who have to share rooms or sleep on one of the many donated couches in Justicia's large living room, Frank and other male volunteers have their own rooms. At various points throughout the day, Frank gets a knock on his door from someone—or a line of people—in need of medicine or other medical resources. The process is straightforward: Frank opens to the door, listens to the men's requests, closes the door, and begins searching through a wide six-foot-high shelf stacked with painkillers, allergy medicine, remedies for an upset stomach, bandages, gauze, rubbing alcohol, and hydrogen peroxide. After locating the needed item, he opens the door and hands it out. For the men, his room operates like one of Houston's smallest and most informal pharmacies.

But the informality of the Third Net is a double-edged sword. On the one hand, spaces like Justicia can directly tend to the needs of migrants legally excluded from the health care system. On the other hand, the labor of providing care falls into the hands of those like Frank who may not be qualified or experienced in tending to a diverse range of medical needs, some of which are very serious and require sustained attention. This is particularly challenging when it comes to mental health. For example, one of the migrant men, Miguel, became suicidal. He told Frank he "didn't want to live anymore" and that he would go back into his room to "end everything." Frank talked to the man for over half an hour before deciding to consult with Margaret, who gave him the green light to call the police and get an ambulance to transport Miguel to Ben Taub for mental health support.

While the men do, of course, confide in one another and provide each other mental and emotional support, they also heavily rely on Frank for this. Frank is less than half the age of Miguel and many of the migrant men at Justicia, and he has no previous social work or mental health training. He is also unfamiliar with evidence-based strategies for mitigating ideas of suicide. Nevertheless, Frank is expected to perform abundant mental and emotional labor: being a confidant for more than 60 men, alleviating arguments, enforcing house rules, and, as in the case of Miguel, talking men out of attempting suicide. Like other Catholic Workers, Frank does whatever he can when mental health emergency situations emerge, but without professional training and experience, he is unable to do much more than listen. This can put volunteers in precarious situations.

For example, Javier, a 21-year-old volunteer, recounts the story of Hector, a Mexican man in his early 20s who struggles to reconcile past traumatic experiences. Most migrants who come to Justicia do so on their own two feet; Hector, by contrast, was carried in, each of his arms wrapped around a different man and both of his legs pierced with bullet holes. Throughout the several weeks he was at the organization, Hector regained the ability to walk and became closer to the other men. Javier recalls the men hugging Hector, saying "you're a part of us; we're your family and friends," and Hector responding, "you guys are friends; you guys are my family." Things seemed to be taking a turn for the better for a while, but then the trauma of past events resurfaced, and no one at Justicia knew how to respond. Javier explains:

> From what I understand, some of his old friends came to pick him up and teased him, saying he wasn't the same gangster as before. They kept teasing him and teasing him, eventually causing him to go into a depression where he started drinking and doing drugs, which Justicia has zero tolerance for. Then one day, I get a call from the men's house saying, "he's inside the bodega—the kitchen." And I go in and see a knife in his hand. So I hug him and put my left hand on his right wrist and twist it to make sure he drops the knife. And then I just keep on hugging him while he cried in my arms. That's when he said, "I have to leave. I don't want to do anything bad to this house." So he got his stuff and left.

The other men could have called Margaret or the police, but instead, they called Javier, a man younger than Hector with zero years of professional mental health experience. While this provides testament to the trust the men have in the volunteers, it simultaneously exhibits a structural deficiency in Justicia's capacity to care. While Javier was able to defuse the situation with Hector, he could have easily been injured or killed.

The challenges associated with mental health extend to the women's house as well. Cynthia, a volunteer, explains: "Many women suffer from debilitating depression, and we're not equipped to deal with that." Several of the women at Justicia came to the organization specifically to escape domestic abuse and various forms of sexual violence. But there is no mental health professional at the clinic for the women to process these experiences, and this serves as a major limitation. Cynthia conveys this with the story of a migrant woman named Berenice:

Maybe a week before Berenice came to Justicia, she had been gang-raped, and her husband witnessed it. A lot of other people witnessed it. She was beaten up, and the bruises were still very, very fresh, and it was one of those cases where Berenice couldn't look at people. She didn't want to be touched. I mean it was really awful, and again, we're not equipped to deal with someone who is that fragile.

Cynthia recognizes mental health as a big challenge at Justicia. While volunteers can refer women to other centers and organizations where they could potentially receive support, they still perform significant mental and emotional labor at Justicia on a daily basis. They do this not because it's their "job"—in fact, not a single volunteer at Justicia characterizes what they do as a job. Rather, they perform this labor because of their personal investment in the women—the Catholic Worker Movement philosophy of personalism requires this level of dedication.

"You think you can be a Catholic Worker by just taking care of the material needs?" asks Sylvia, a volunteer. "No way. It's more much personal than that." She explains:

Like for instance, [some other Catholic Workers and I] were in the middle of a movie and [a migrant woman named Valeria] came and knocked on the door. So I left the room to talk to her and she just like broke down and wept. She was having some huge marital issue and considering divorce and like, she's like 40-something and I'm like 20. I'm like out of high school, and like I don't have any wisdom on marriage. Lord. [*laughs*] And so we sat and talked, and basically I had to talk to her for like an hour before she was peaceful enough to go back to bed.

Valeria could have reached out to any of the other migrant women at Justicia closer to her age or someone who had been married before, but instead she decided to confide in Sylvia, a woman half her age with no marriage experience. While Sylvia is happy to provide support, she recognizes the limits of her knowledge and experiences: "You find yourself being confided in, and like the whole time and you feel totally inadequate. When Valeria talked to me, I was just standing there thinking, 'do you realize that I'm like younger than all your children?'"

Third Net practitioners like Sylvia offer more than just material support. They also provide a level of emotional support that often goes beyond their personal and professional experience. Reminiscent of other migrants who turn to volunteers for support, Valeria's decision to go to Sylvia is significant because it illustrates a particular type of trust between migrants and Catholic Workers that may be more difficult to establish in formal settings. In hospitals and clinics, health practitioners are trusted as medical experts, those who can accurately evaluate and address biomedical ailments. In Third Net spaces like Justicia, practitioners are entrusted to be jacks-of-all-trades—that is, non-expert experts of various areas like medicine, mental health, family dynamics, and more.

Migrants Remain at the Bottom of the Organization Hierarchy

Of course, every Third Net space is structured differently, but at Justicia, migrants remain at the bottom of the organizational hierarchy. Philosophically, Catholic Worker–inspired spaces like Justicia are supposed to be structured in ways that allow everyone to chime in about how to manifest Christ's teachings; that is, everyone should have a say on what care entails at Justicia.[81] In practice, however, everyone has a distinct location on Justicia's hierarchical ladder (figure 2.2): Margaret and her late husband Larry sit at the top, followed by volunteers, the men's house manager (Jose), Jose's 14 "helpers," and then all other migrants at Justicia. The central consequence of this organizational hierarchy is that it reifies a social hierarchy wherein migrants are allotted the least agency in dictating what immigrant justice looks like.

With Larry's passing, Margaret serves as Justicia's prime director. While she routinely confers with an informal board of other select volunteers (those with years of experience at Justicia), she ultimately makes final decisions. Several volunteers note that this can create challenges for organizational stability. For example, nothing in the clinic is digitized— hundreds of patient files are stored in hardcopy form and continue to occupy more and more space over time. Despite volunteers' suggestions, Margaret adamantly rejects the notion of digitizing these files, expressing concern over the information leaking out or being digitally lost (e.g., if the storage device becomes corrupt and unusable). These concerns

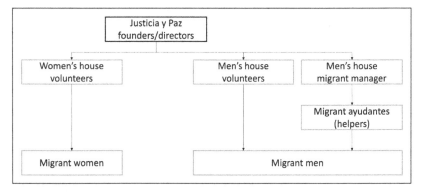

Figure 2.2. Justicia y Paz organizational hierarchy

are understandable, considering that every person who uses the clinic is undocumented, and of course, Margaret wants to do everything in her power to protect migrants' identities and lives. Still, Margaret's authority is readily visible and reminiscent of other houses of hospitality in the US. Caleb, a volunteer, shares that he has lived in several houses of hospitality across the country, including San Antonio, Des Moines, San Francisco, Denver, and New Orleans. While discussing varying structures of the organizations he has volunteered with, Caleb shared, "It's an interesting phenomenon because in some situations, they're almost like little dictatorships because Larry and Margaret make every decision when it comes to finances and who gets helped. Not that they don't listen to other people. They are open to suggestions, but it's really their baby, and they run it. And I think that's typical." Although Caleb noted that Justicia Directors Larry and Margaret were "open to suggestions," his characterization of houses of hospitality as "little dictatorships" reflects the widely shared sentiment that they ultimately have the final say on how things go.

Volunteers and migrants alike share reservations about Margaret's authority. While many migrants express appreciation for Margaret and Justicia as a whole, some report feeling unable to voice new ideas or criticisms about the organization. Manuel, a migrant, summarizes: "Margaret doesn't listen to others. It's like this or like that. That's all." Elias, an older Mexican man in his late 70s, echoes this sentiment. When asked if there were any problems at Justicia, he responded, "Yes, if you speak up."

When probed for more information he continued, "I just told you. If we speak up, there's trouble. Do you want me to get in trouble? If you see something you shut your mouth. The rules are already made up, and if you don't like them, you're free to leave. They won't ask anyone to stay." Margaret does meet with migrants at the men's house on a weekly basis to see how things are going, but, as both Manuel and Elias convey, it's difficult to put new ideas into motion.

While volunteers generally have to go through Margaret to facilitate changes to the organization itself, they wield significant autonomy when it comes to completing day-to-day activities at Justicia. This is largely because every day looks different and comes with its own set of challenges and tasks. While volunteers' day-to-day responsibilities vary, they constantly remain migrants' go-to for everything. Sylvia, a volunteer, explains:

> [Migrant guests] have to ask me for everything from medicine and supplies to information about everything. . . . If I vomit in the middle of the night, I can go find myself medicine or go get the car and drive to get medical help if I need it, you know what I mean? They don't have any of that. They have to come to us [volunteers] for all of it, even just a pill for a headache or oil to cook dinner. Everything. It's really [*pauses to think*]. In some ways it really is comparable to like a parenting thing.

While volunteers have the agency to obtain resources from the organization whenever necessary, migrant guests have to go through volunteers to obtain these same resources—a setup that Sylvia characterizes as infantilizing. This paternalistic framework sets up the expectation/assumption that migrants are unable or not trustworthy enough to care for themselves. For example, volunteers at the women's house sort through hundreds of donated clothes every day and then later hand them out to migrant women in a systematic, organized way. When asked why volunteers don't just allow the women to choose which clothes they want and then bag the remaining donations, Sylvia responds, "Oh my gosh, can you imagine? That would be a disaster!" She explained that the women would become "like children" and fight over clothes, much like kids would fight over toys. At the men's house, migrants similarly have to go through Frank for things like medicine and clothing.

When it comes to migrants' power, things differ between the women's house and men's house. At the women's house, migrant women have to ask volunteers for everything and are assigned one of three tasks—cooking, cleaning, and taking out the trash—throughout the week. Here, volunteers manage all day-to-day activities. The men's house is a little different because there are so many men there at one time (generally more than 60). At the men's house, volunteers wield the most power, followed by Jose (the men's house manager), the ayudantes (helpers), and then the rest of the migrant men. Jose, a Mexican man in his late 30s, lives at the men's house and manages all day-to-day activities. He can decide not only who gets admitted into the men's house, but also who has to leave. If other men disrespect the rules of the house, he can ask them to leave or call the police to have them forcibly removed. Though volunteers like Frank hold more power than Jose, they generally defer to Jose's decisions. Frank says, "In terms of making decisions, I generally just go to Jose because he usually has really good answers and more experience." Jose also routinely bounces ideas off of Frank and other volunteers. The only person Jose is beholden to is Margaret. At times, Jose shares, this can be stifling: "I want to help people and it breaks my heart that I can't. It feels awful when someone needs help and I can't help them because [Margaret] wouldn't let me, but I respect that. I understand her position, you know, she's the owner."[82] Jose links explicitly to language that places Margaret at the top of the hierarchy and migrants at the bottom. Observing Jose and Margaret's interactions, Jose's body language also suggests deference. Whenever Margaret walks into the room, he always immediately perks up, stands up straight, and crosses his hands behind his back. Reflecting on these non-verbal cues, Manuel characterizes Jose as a direct subordinate of Margaret's: "Jose is like Margaret's soldier."

Because there are so many people at the men's house, Jose chooses 14 other migrant men to serve as his ayudantes. Chosen by Jose on the basis of work ethic and dedication to Justicia's mission, the 14 men primarily rotate two tasks: cooking and serving as door attendants. Every day of the week, a different ayudante is responsible for cooking lunch and dinner. Meals vary widely and depend entirely on what has been donated to the organization. Door attendants manage who comes in and out of the men's house, and when a new person arrives they are responsible for checking the individual in and familiarizing them with the house's rules, activities, and expectations. Each of the 14 ayudantes is also in charge of one of the 12 different bedrooms at the men's house, making sure that each room's six to eight guests follow the rules and get what they need. All of the ayudantes' decisions go through Jose, who ultimately reports to Margaret about how things are going. While Jose and the ayudantes enjoy certain benefits like being able to get themselves food from the kitchen or stay up past the 10 p.m. curfew, other migrant men have to ask ayudantes, Jose, or volunteers for everything.

As one volunteer put it, the structure of Justicia is very "top-down." In practical terms, such a hierarchical structure facilitates a degree of organizational control, but in social terms, this reifies the very forms of social control Catholic Worker philosophy rejects. Taking stock of the disproportionate decision-making power at Justicia may help spaces similar to Justicia create further opportunities for migrant-volunteer collaboration, allyship, and immigrant justice solidarity.

The Linchpin of Justicia's Internal Infrastructure: "The Suffering Migrant"

The postal codes stamped onto Justicia's newsletters range from the Houston metropolitan region to the Vatican City, providing testament to the sheer scale of support the organization receives. On top of this, Justicia receives clothes and furniture donations every single day of the year. Kiara, a volunteer, shares that when people drop off donations, they frequently say things like "I wanted to donate to a Catholic house" or "I just wanted to give back to immigrants and the Hispanic community" or, for the most part, "I just wanted to donate to a good organization with a good cause."

The image of "the suffering migrant" is pervasive and powerful within the Catholic Worker Movement. Most pages of the organization's news-letter spotlight migrants' dire experiences. As noted earlier in the chapter, volunteers like Henry regularly draw on the image of suffering to highlight the Catholic Worker Movement's impact: "Think of all the upper-class people who wouldn't otherwise be donating and thinking about the poor and suffering immigrant and not having an opportunity to participate and alleviate that suffering." When appealing to church pa-rishioners for organizational support, Catholic Workers routinely invoke the movement's philosophy about serving Christ through serving the poor. The public absorbs narratives about the "suffering migrant" and "deserving poor" so repeatedly that the two become entwined with one another. The image of the "suffering migrant" inspires empathy, compassion, and movement—the movement of goods, resources, and labor. It propels the movement of money, medical supplies, food, furniture, and volunteer labor throughout Justicia's internal infrastructure; it's the narrative that compels Harris Health doctors to volunteer their time, and it's the reason hundreds of people put checks made out to Justicia in the mail every year. The image of the "suffering migrant" serves as the linchpin of Justicia's entire internal infrastructure, which means that within Justicia, migrants are unable to fully transcend the role and identity of the "suffering migrant." In other words, they are stripped of their agency to "not suffer" and racialized as in perpetual need of "saving."[83]

The perpetuity of migrants' "suffering" condition can be understood in relation to the Bible's Gospel of Matthew, which inspires Catholic Worker Movement philosophy and all of Justicia's activities. Referencing Matthew 25, Margaret explains, "The Lord in the disguise of the poor who comes to us—that's what it's all about. It's the whole meaning of what we do." Further, in Matthew 26, verse 11, Jesus says "you always have the poor with you," a line which, according to theologian Rachel Muers, divinely eternalizes both the condition of poverty itself and the notion that some moral, privileged group is to be responsible for addressing it.[84] Thus, power distinctions between Catholic Worker practitioners/supporters and migrants at Justicia are both permanent and divinely sanctioned. Volunteers, church practitioners, doctors, social workers, food bank administrators, and everyday ordinary citizens who donate to Justicia play the "savior" role; they all participate in the grand Catholic Worker project of "service to the poor." Migrants, on the other hand, play the perpetual role of the always in need, always suffering "deserving poor." Like other "disempowered populations" across other Catholic Worker sites,[85] migrants' deservingness hinges on the image of suffering.

Can Catholic Workers get behind the project of migrant justice *without* conceptualizing migrants as needy and dependent? In other words, can Catholic Worker–inspired spaces like Justicia exist *without* the "suffering migrant"? If not, then "service to the poor" becomes the same type of charity work that spaces like Justicia attempt to reject—that is, where the powerful (Catholic Workers) simply give to the purportedly powerless (migrants).

Third Net spaces like Justicia are well intentioned and undoubtedly instrumental in the lives of migrants who find themselves excluded from the formal tiers of our health care system. Indeed, the spiritual revolution of the heart that Dorothy Day and Peter Maurin envisioned at the genesis of the Catholic Worker Movement fundamentally involves learning to see one another as human beings. But one's humanity cannot simply be visible under the limelight of indigence. Pain and suffering are not the only things that make us human and are problematic bases on which to inspire social movement support. The image of the "suffering migrant" is highly influential, in part for its power to anoint some as saviors. As later chapters attest, it is not the only ideology that can drive collective action.

Conclusion

Everything culminates at the Third Net, and this is intentional. Rome was deliberately positioned such that no matter which road was taken, the Roman Empire was centered; hence the famous aphorism "all roads lead to Rome." When it comes to low-income undocumented migrants in need of care (medical provisions, food, shelter, etc.), all roads lead to the Third Net—that is, spaces like Justicia. Unlike Rome, however, the Third Net is not the locus or metropole of power. Instead, it is a dumping ground. The health care system is not made up of cracks and fractures; it is purposively designed to exclude low-income undocumented migrants and ultimately direct them to informal Third Net spaces like Justicia. Physicians, medical social workers, health care navigators, and hospital staff all turn to Justicia for health care delivery. At the same time, Justicia mobilizes an enormous pool of human and material resources ranging from a relatively steady stream of volunteer labor to millions of dollars of support every year.

The case of Justicia illustrates how broad the Third Net is. While all the work Justicia does is amazing, it is equally alarming. Volunteer doctors address medical conditions at Justicia precisely because these conditions are not addressed in the formal sectors of the health care system. Private residents and migrant families pick up the work of informal home care because formal institutions of long-term care (e.g., nursing homes) are exorbitantly expensive and inaccessible. Migrants come to Justicia for food, clothing, and shelter because it is nearly impossible to make a livable wage, and other social institutions offer little recourse. The reason all roads lead to the Third Net is because it's the only terrain left when other health care and social safety nets deteriorate, and they're still deteriorating. All presidents—whether Democrat or Republican—have continued to expand the Reagan-era legacy of privatized medicine.[86] Such privatization means the continual withering away of the formal health care safety net and fewer health care options for both undocumented migrants and indigent citizens in the midst of increasing housing precarity[87] and food insecurity.[88]

Both citizens and noncitizens recurrently find themselves legally excluded from an assortment of institutions (e.g., education, employment, housing, health care). Consequently, the Third Net emerges as a last resort for potentially everyone. Justicia dedicates all of its time and resources to addressing migrants' various medical and social needs, but across the globe, other Catholic Worker–inspired houses of hospitality focus on the needs of indigent citizens. Third Net spaces like Justicia survive because they have extensive internal infrastructures of support. Though there are limitations to Justicia's Catholic Worker–inspired philosophy of the "deserving poor," it is nonetheless compelling and draws in tremendous support from literally thousands of people across the greater Houston metropolitan region and the globe. Doctors from the Harris Health System make it possible for Justicia to provide migrants primary care. Private residents and migrant families provide limited albeit important home care to migrants in need of long-term care. The food bank and local churches enable the organization to feed hundreds of people every week. Universities offer Justicia a stream of volunteers eager to meet migrants' diverse needs. And members of the wider community who donate money, clothes, and furniture to Justicia facilitate the organization's ability to continue its day-to-day operations. Like other Third Net spaces, Justicia's material/symbolic resources go to transform a basket of a few fishes and loaves of bread into a cache of medical supplies, food, and provisions.

In the next chapter, we shift our attention to the work of CommUnity Clinic of Phoenix, a free migrant-serving clinic that condemns charity models of care and promotes a systemic understanding of "immigrant health justice."

3

Beyond Charity

The back door opens to vivid colors and cacophonous chatter. The small orange kitchen with bright Spanish tile countertops is overflowing with volunteers as usual. The room, which also operates as a back office, supply room, break room, and general volunteer hangout space, is bursting with boxes of medical supplies, volunteers' backpacks, piles of T-shirts emblazoned with the clinic's logo, and secondhand scrubs for sale. A large dog bed is occupied by the golden retriever therapy dog that makes regular trips out to the waiting room to visit patients. Volunteer nurses and medical providers in scrubs with stethoscopes around their necks occupy the seats at the long folding table that takes up the entire kitchen space. They all have laptops open in front of them reviewing the appointment schedule, catching up on patient files, and talking across the table together about who would see which patients that day.

"Sonia, how about you do her H&P?" Michael shouts from one end of the long table to Sonia, a nursing volunteer sitting at the other end. "I'll send her back to the lab now to go ahead and get her bloodwork done. I want to make sure that she sees Alondra before she leaves here today." The two are coordinating care for a new patient, Juanita, who arrived at the clinic this morning. At a patient's first visit, they get an H&P, or medical history and full physical. For the clinic's patients, this includes bloodwork, urinalysis, EKG, and, if the patient has diabetes, examinations for wounds on their feet and tests for neuropathy. Often this is the first time a patient has had medical care in years.

Around the table of medical providers, intake and lab volunteers and holistic services practitioners who don't need to be on the computer or who arrived too late to get a spot at the table hover around the periphery of the kitchen, making it impossible to move around the room without squishing between and around volunteers. Newly arrived volunteers have to step on people's toes, muttering apologies, as they make their way to the large alphabetized file to retrieve their volunteer ID and scan the barcode to sign in. They tiptoe around the obstacle course of the kitchen, careful not to knock over Alondra's rain sticks leaning in the corner or kick her singing bowl.

Beyond the bright orange kitchen crammed with volunteers, what was originally a living room with a huge fireplace covered in Spanish tile now functions as the waiting room with a small folding table where intake volunteers sign in patients for their appointments and take their information. Three cramped bedrooms operate as exam rooms, with one reserved for holistic services, midwifery, and women's health appointments. A fourth tiny bedroom with walk-in closet and bathroom comprise the makeshift lab and biomedical and naturopathic pharmacy, where patients have their blood drawn and leave with glucometers, lancets, and blood sugar testing strips or vitamins, supplements, and homeopathic remedies.

Back in the lab, Juanita sits in the phlebotomy chair, one sleeve of her shirt rolled up above her elbow, waiting to get her blood drawn. Juanita is an "emergency" patient, which at CommUnity Clinic of Phoenix[1] means a patient with underlying chronic yet treatable medical conditions that have gone untreated, usually for years. Juanita is a mother from Mexico who has been recently widowed; her eyesight has begun to deteriorate rapidly—an indication of prolonged, uncontrolled diabetes—and she is now legally blind. Her health condition also affects her ability to work, and as a result, her family is facing serious financial struggles on top of these health issues. In the absence of health care, CommUnity volunteers worry that her high blood pressure and uncontrolled diabetes will jeopardize her kidneys' function or even put her life in danger. During this first appointment, volunteers hope to get a better sense not only of the extent of Juanita's physical health issues but also of the larger context of her life situation as it affects her mental and physical health.

Most new patients at the clinic are quiet and at least a little nervous in the clinic before they get to know the volunteers and became more comfortable, but Juanita cracks jokes throughout her first appointment despite the seriousness of her health condition. As the lab assistant searches for a vein in her arm to draw vials of blood for her initial lab work, she jokes that they can't find one because she is too fat. Despite the seriousness of her high blood pressure and the uncontrolled diabetes progressed to the point that it is affecting her eyesight, Juanita has the lab filled with laughter.

In all first appointments at CommUnity, new patients receive most of the usual lab work and physical examinations they would get at a primary care physician, but unlike a doctor's visit in the mainstream health system, these initial appointments also include visits with the holistic care providers at the clinic. Before Juanita leaves the clinic, she will also have appointments with the clinic's mental health counselor, Octavia, and the volunteer curandera, Alondra, who uses indigenous and spiritual healing practices like sound healing and feather work with the clinic's patients. As Juanita meets with Alondra, the sound of the crystal singing bowl and Alondra's chanting reverberates around the tiny clinic space.

* * *

Located in a small, nondescript house on a busy corner in central Phoenix, CommUnity Clinic of Phoenix (CommUnity or CCP for short) is a free clinic for uninsured patients, mainly undocumented Latinx migrants like Juanita. Unlicensed and underground with no sign on the outside of the house, the clinic operates under the radar to protect the identity of its patients. But, for the communities that it serves and the nonprofit organizations and medical providers who refer patients to the clinic, CommUnity's existence and services are very much a "known secret."[2] This secrecy is in part a result of Arizona's notorious immigration enforcement policies that create a culture of surveillance and criminalization for undocumented migrants in the state. Migrants avoid accessing medical care in the mainstream health system for fear of encountering law enforcement and being detected as undocumented.[3]

This secrecy also underscores the Third Net's operations in an informal, and sometimes underground, health care infrastructure.[4] Free clinics and NGOs in the Third Net assume a variety of approaches to migrant health care provision (some of which were discussed in chapter 1) that often map onto debates about charity versus justice approaches to social service provision and community organizing.[5] A charity model of migrant health care usually emphasizes meeting immediate health needs for as many patients as possible. Often working tirelessly with limited resources, the majority of free clinics and charities can only provide the bare minimum in terms of primary care, including limited health screenings and access to some medications. In the absence of health care access for their patients in the formal system, these charities and free clinics are often characterized as providing a "band-aid" approach and, with shoe-string budgets juxtaposed with exorbitant costs of medical services in the US, "suffer systemically from inferior quality."[6]

Working within these same material constraints, CommUnity takes a different approach to care predicated on their vision and commitment to "immigrant health justice."[7] This approach involves an important distinction from charity models in both discourse and practice. Immigrant health justice involves an indictment of the structural failures of the immigration and health systems that recognizes the ill health and premature deaths of uninsured, undocumented migrants as results of the problems inherent in these systems. This critique spurs action. Immigrant health justice in practice focuses on providing quality personalized care to patients, while working to build a movement for health justice and migrant rights.

CommUnity's work demonstrates the capacity of the Third Net to challenge charity models of migrant health care. It is their vision and practice of immigrant health justice that represents a direct challenge to the systemic failures of the immigration and health systems in the US as well as charity models of free health care. Marked by a commitment to quality care, immigrant health justice frames health care provision for uninsured, undocumented migrants as strategic political advocacy amid a culture of migrant exclusion and criminalization.[8] It works to recast migrant patients outside the anti-immigrant rhetoric and popular discourses of dependency, (un)deservingness, and suffering. In practice, the structural constraints and limited resources of current immigration and health systems pose challenges to CommUnity's radical vision of health care for all regardless of income, insurance, or immigration status. As a result, CommUnity must navigate a host of interorganizational infrastructural challenges and interpersonal tensions. The clinic works to address these challenges, in part, through combining a variety of seemingly contradictory approaches to health—Western biomedicine, naturopathic medicine, and holistic and spiritual healing practices—to create a collage of care for the clinic's patients.

This chapter begins with an examination of the clinic's history, mission, and vision of migrant health justice[9] that sets the clinic's work apart from charity models of care in the Third Net. Next, it outlines the internal and external challenges that CommUnity faces in achieving this radical vision of migrant health justice, as it works to navigate the persistent structural constraints of the current immigration and health systems. Finally, it discusses the "collage of care" created by the complementary relationship among the various health approaches at the clinic: Western biomedicine, naturopathic medicine, and holistic and spiritual healing techniques. Together, these approaches fashion a patchwork of healing services that forms the personalized, quality care that CommUnity provides its patients. Chapter 2 discussed the vital work of Justicia y Paz and what Third Net organizations are able to accomplish with little resources and informal infrastructure. This chapter focuses on the critique of the mainstream health system and health care infrastructure produced by Third Net organizations, through examining the discourse and practice of CommUnity. CommUnity and Justicia share many commonalities as social justice–focused organizations working in the Third Net to provide health care to uninsured, undocumented migrants. Whereas Justicia provides temporary shelter, food, and other social services in addition to medical care in the vein of a Catholic Worker house, CommUnity is primarily a free clinic, premised on the principles of both the migrant rights movement that asserts "no one is illegal" and health justice movements that argue for the right to free health care for all.

Clinic History: From a "Guerrilla Clinic" to a "Clinic with Walls"

CommUnity's origin story is centered not in charity medical provision or religious imperatives, but in political protest. The clinic was begun by members of Metro Area Street Health (MASH),[10] a group of street medics that provided water and medical attention to dehydrated, tear-gassed protesters at migrant rights actions in Phoenix. Around 2010, the group coalesced into a more organized collective after a series of protests around Arizona's infamous SB 1070 legislation.[11] At one protest in particular, the police shot hundreds of rubber bullets into the crowd and indiscriminately tear-gassed protesters. MASH volunteers treated toddlers in strollers, pregnant women, elderly people, and others who were victims of the police's use of force.

After the passage of SB 1070,[12] migrants increasingly avoided public spaces, and even formal health care settings, for fear of encounters with law enforcement or detection as undocumented. In a documentary film about the clinic's work,[13] Michael, a registered nurse and one of the founders of both MASH and CommUnity, recalled the care they were able to provide for people who would otherwise have gone without medical services:

> After SB 1070 passed, our immigrant neighbors started to feel more and more afraid to engage with formal health settings and other official organizations in the city. They were too afraid to go to the doctor or the emergency room. Some folks wouldn't even leave their homes. It's hard to relate the culture of fear in Phoenix at the time. Those of us in the MASH collective started to get calls from people that weren't related to the protests. In these calls, folks would say things like, "My baby is sick with a fever. Can someone come look at her?" or, "My husband has had diarrhea for four days. He's too weak to get out of bed." This wasn't something we had expected, but we responded as best we could.

Drawing on their links within the migrant community in Phoenix, MASH created an informal network of patients and health care provision that constituted what the collective members described as a "guerilla clinic," going practically door-to-door to meet patients in their homes. Michael discussed this history, waxing nostalgic about the early days when MASH members began to provide more informal health care: "Those early days when we started doing house calls, we drove around Phoenix to people's homes to check on them. I like to say that we were a guerrilla clinic. Thinking back to that time, in hindsight, it's amazing to me how much we were able to do without a formal clinic. We were just a few friends with medical training and supplies we carried around in our cars and backpacks." Lorena, another MASH member who became a founder of CommUnity, described these origins as "always unapologetically activist."

As the demand for home visits increased, MASH volunteers eventually purchased and renovated a decrepit private home as a clinic space filled with donated medical equipment. Ed, a physician assistant and MASH and CCP volunteer, described this transition as moving from a "guerrilla clinic" to a "clinic with walls." Although the collective was able to accomplish much with little formal organization or resources, the new clinic space drastically increased the capacity of the MASH collective to provide care for uninsured, undocumented migrants who were largely ineligible for and afraid to access health care in the formal system.

As CommUnity grew and received more patient referrals by word of mouth or from local migrant rights organizations, financial resources—in particular the lab costs associated with patients' blood work—remained the primary constraint on the number of patients CCP could take on. As a health care provider in the Third Net, CommUnity receives no government or grant funding, relying almost entirely on individual donations to operate. These donations range from a few dollars that patients put in the donation jar at the clinic to substantial financial investments from a couple of wealthy benefactors. In a herculean effort, CCP volunteers devote countless hours to organizing fundraising events, including art shows, pig roasts, film screenings, and drag shows, to raise awareness and money for the clinic. However, there is a noticeable feeling of futility in selling stickers, T-shirts, mugs, and secondhand scrubs for what feels like spare change compared to a single patient's ER bills that can run into the tens of thousands of dollars. But CommUnity is able to cobble together the funds it needs to keep the lights on, so to speak, and ensure that patients have access to free health care and medications. In its refusal to apply for government or foundation grant funding, CCP has an approach to fundraising similar to Justicia's discussed in the previous chapter. Both organizations rely primarily on individual donations to keep their organizations running, a feat that requires a large volunteer and donor base, targeted publicity of the organization's work to potential donors, and fundraising campaigns that require considerable volunteer time and effort. Many Third Net organizations like Justicia and CommUnity have chosen to forgo government and foundation grant funding in order to maintain certain levels of anonymity from more official channels for the sake of their work and patients as well as to maintain organizational independence from the perceived and real "strings attached" to this funding that may force the organization to shift its programming priorities or that are seen to be at odds with the organizations' mission and goals.

In addition to its dependency on fundraising efforts, CommUnity relies on donations of cast-off equipment from local medical practices. In fact, the entire clinic is furnished with donated medical equipment. This donated equipment—often outdated and sometimes still functional—ensures that patients can receive health services, like EKGs, in house at no cost. However, sometimes these donations can be more trouble than help. For instance, one of the three small exam rooms in the clinic was dominated by an old ophthalmology exam chair, a metal dinosaur of a machine donated by a local eye doctor. A team of muscular EMTs who volunteer at CCP removed what was an extremely heavy and unwieldy piece of medical equipment from the ophthalmologist's office to make room for a new exam chair for his paying patients. CCP organizers kept the nonfunctional equipment, in hopes that they would eventually find a volunteer who could fix it and then could provide eye care to their patients. Routine eye exams for people with uncontrolled diabetes are incredibly important, as prolonged high blood sugar levels can cause retina damage and other eye issues, but eye care for uninsured, low-income patients is often prohibitively expensive and one of the services that is particularly difficult to access for uninsured patients. Had the clinic ever gotten this equipment to work, then diabetic patients like Juanita with deteriorating eyesight would have had access to free eye exams. But for CCP, this vision remained an unrealized dream. The only beneficiary of this old exam chair was the ophthalmologist who donated it to the clinic—he was able to write the donation off as a tax break, even though the equipment was nonfunctional. In this way, the Third Net's members not only accommodate the *people* who are cast off by the mainstream health care system and provide care for them, but they also accommodate *things* cast off by it—trying to refurbish and make do with outdated medical equipment that would often be better suited for a landfill. And in this way, they provide additional financial incentives and support to the mainstream health system through tax write-offs. CommUnity would have been better served by this same doctor providing pro bono appointments with the clinic's most vulnerable patients.

Because of the ad hoc nature and informality of the Third Net, free clinics and nonprofits rely on expansive networks for donations (i.e., money and equipment) and pro bono specialist care. This reliance on networks in the community as well as within the formal health system necessitates a large, well-connected volunteer base. Given the demands of the formal clinic space, CommUnity's transition to a "clinic with walls" generated an influx of new volunteers, including a large number of young, white aspiring health professionals from the suburbs who were looking for experience working with an "underserved community" as a way to boost their prospects of admission to physician assistant and medical schools. These new volunteers were not connected to the MASH collective or the migrant rights movement nor rooted in local migrant communities, and so did not share the experiences or perspective on migrant health care of the clinic's founders. As a result, the original MASH members and core CCP volunteers engaged in regular trainings for volunteers in immigration policy and migrant experiences. Perhaps more important was the regular, significant discursive work performed by clinic founders who sought to educate new CommUnity volunteers about the organization's mission and vision of migrant health care. In this way, the core CCP board members and founders challenge assumptions about the nature of their work as charity or service by explicitly framing the clinic's mission and health care provision as political advocacy.[14]

Clinic Mission: "Not a Free Version of a Broken System"

Fundamental to the discursive framing of the clinic's approach to migrant health care is an assessment of the structural failures of immigration and health policies in the US as well as the limitations of a charity model of migrant care. These critiques shape CommUnity's mission, which in turn informs how volunteers interact with their patients and how medical services are allocated and provided at the clinic. Centering a politicized assessment of migrant health care, CommUnity endeavors to create a model of health care provision that is "not a free version of a broken system," a phrase repeated around the clinic like a mantra. Although it's a seemingly simple phrase, this mission is multi-layered and complex: on the one hand, it encapsulates the clinic's analysis of the brokenness of immigration and health care systems in the US, while on the other hand, it involves the implicit critique of other forms of free health care provision that they consider to replicate the structural failures of immigrant health care. In this way, CommUnity defines itself and its work not only against the larger systems of immigration and health, but also against other forms of charity care.

Informing the clinic's approach, CommUnity's critique of migrant health care in the US involves a three-pronged analysis of the inherent problems with this system. First, CCP takes aim at the exclusionary, privatized nature of health care provision in the US, which prevents a large swath of the population from accessing medical care in the mainstream health system, including people who cannot afford health insurance or medical services as well as those who are ineligible for health care coverage, specifically undocumented migrants. According to clinic organizers, the for-profit nature of the mainstream health system is a fundamental aspect of its "brokenness." Cheryl, a nurse and long-time CommUnity volunteer, described this critique to new volunteers on a Thursday clinic day, saying,

> The health system is inherently broken on a structural level . . . I mean, it's a health system, is it not supposed to make people healthy? But there is no way we could argue that we are getting healthier on the whole . . . the system isn't working for people because it's looking for customers and consumers. At CCP, we are working to ensure that we do not simply replicate a free version of this broken system.

Cheryl's statement, echoed by all clinic founders and core volunteers, draws attention to the paradoxical nature of the privatized health system in the US. Arguing that health care should never be associated with a profit motive, Donna, one of the main clinic organizers, would regularly comment that the deteriorated health of the clinic's patients and the ever-increasing costs of medical services and medications were "evidence that people's health should not be a business." CCP organizers assert that medical care designed to function as a profit-making enterprise leads to the denial of health care to patients who cannot afford it. This profit motive, combined with anti-immigrant sentiment and policies, produces a class of "non-patients" excluded from or ineligible for health care due to their socioeconomic or immigration status.

This critique of the for-profit health system extends to the current health care policies that were dictated by the Affordable Care Act (ACA). Unlike Texas, Arizona expanded Medicaid under the ACA, thus raising the income threshold for eligibility so that an additional 500,000 previously uninsured residents qualified for health coverage. When asked about the legislation's impact for CommUnity patients, Michael described the benefits and limitations of the ACA:

> The ACA provided coverage for a whole lot of people in Arizona who weren't insured before, and that's important. I'm not going to pretend like it's not important. Those people have health care access now. But the issue with the ACA is that it only expanded an already broken system. It provides privatized, for-profit health care to more US citizens. It didn't address the fundamental brokenness of the system.

Arguing that the ACA is a mere expansion of the existing problematic health system in the US, Michael points to the continued exclusion of non-citizens (and a considerable number of citizens as well) who remain unable to get health coverage under the policy. As the remaining uninsured population in states that expanded Medicaid is largely unauthorized migrants, the ACA has actually widened the gulf in health disparities between insured US citizens and uninsured migrants. In the midst of their continued exclusion from health coverage, the only recourse for medical care for uninsured migrants is either in hospital emergency rooms or in Third Net sites, like CommUnity, that provide limited services.

Second, in addition to the for-profit, private health system that denies medical care to those in the most need, the organizers at CommUnity take aim at the US immigration system. Especially in the context of local Arizona politics, CommUnity volunteers call out the surveillance and criminalization of Latinx and migrant communities through policies like SB 1070. They link this anti-immigrant rhetoric and legislation directly to a "broken" immigration system with few avenues for migrants to access authorized status. During a training on immigration policy, Nayeli, a former CommUnity patient and immigrant rights activist who worked for the local ACLU chapter, educated new volunteers to better understand the experiences of the clinic's patients. Discussing the state's immigration legislation, Nayeli said,

> Arizona is notorious for its harsh immigration policies that force immigrants to live in fear, to live in the shadows. We've all heard a lot about SB 1070, but it is just one of the most recent policies in a long line of legislation that denies the rights of immigrants in this state, from denying young people in-state tuition at local colleges to keeping people from getting driver's licenses. [Sheriff] Arpaio famously said that he could tell an undocumented immigrant just by looking at their shoes, and he used to have large U-Haul-sized MCSO [Maricopa County Sheriff's Office] trucks that said on the side, "Call this number to report illegal aliens." It was basically a deportation hotline. Can you imagine all of this stress? Can you imagine what it would be like to be someone without status in this environment? We want to view this issue not through the criminal justice system, but through the lens of the desperation of immigrant workers who are trying to make a better life for their family.

In this discussion and throughout the workshop, Nayeli highlighted the confluence of federal and local immigration policies that kept migrants (and CCP patients) from being able to access authorized status. She also reframed the debate from focusing on the "criminal justice system," including what she described as "the criminalizing rhetoric that brands immigrants as illegal," instead emphasizing the perspective of migrants themselves. By centering migrants' disenfranchisement, CCP critiques immigration policies and enforcement tactics as creating a culture of fear, forcing migrants to live "in the shadows," and exacerbating migrant health disparities. This culture of fear and surveillance makes health care even more inaccessible for many Latinx and migrant communities.

Lastly, beyond the brokenness of these singular systems, CCP argues that mainstream health care and immigration enforcement have intersecting and compounding effects for undocumented migrants needing health care in the US. In a workshop for new volunteers on the clinic's vision of migrant health care, Ed, another clinic founder and physician assistant, explained:

In thinking about what our own patients have gone through when trying to access health care, it's important to remember that Arpaio and his
goons used to park their trucks and sit outside the ER, checking people's
papers as they went into the hospital. . . . They would turn up at free
health fairs put on for the [Latinx migrant] community and round people
up. We need to be aware of this because for new patients walking into
the clinic, this is the history of health care access in this state that they
have as their frame of reference. It's a scary situation. And it's no wonder
that many of them haven't tried to get medical care in the formal health
system.

In this discussion, Ed recounts the immigration enforcement tactics
that specifically target surveillance at migrants trying to access health
care, either in the hospital emergency room or through community
health fairs designed to provide basic health screenings for uninsured
people. Ed directly connects health care and immigration enforcement
tactics, describing how the fear of immigration enforcement dampens
health-seeking behavior for migrants in the US and renders even emergency medical care inaccessible. In this context, accessing public sector
services like health care can be just as dangerous for undocumented
migrants as being stopped for a broken taillight.

As a result, CommUnity's patients would often refuse to go to the
emergency room when they were experiencing a serious health crisis
that the clinic was ill equipped to manage. For instance, Juanita, the
young single mother with untreated high blood pressure and uncontrolled diabetes at the beginning of the chapter, ended up having a
stroke as a result of her medical conditions going untreated for years.
Despite the urgings of the volunteers at CommUnity, she refused to go
to the emergency room for fear of being apprehended by immigration
enforcement or turned over to immigration enforcement by hospital officials. Other studies have documented the ubiquity of this health care
avoidance by uninsured, undocumented migrants across the country.[15]
The real or perceived collusion between immigration enforcement and
medical professionals in the mainstream health system has dire consequences for migrant health and effectively makes emergency medical
care—the only care to which uninsured, undocumented migrants remain eligible—virtually inaccessible.

Contrast with Charity Models of Care

In addition to these systemic challenges, CommUnity's resistance to replicating "a free version of a broken system" involves a critique of dominant approaches to charity health care. As noted earlier, within the Third Net, there is variation among organizations in their approaches to providing health services to uninsured, undocumented migrants. According to CommUnity volunteers, many of these organizations replicate the patient-provider interactions of the mainstream health system and do little to challenge or address the deeper structural causes of migrant health disparities. These free clinics are often characterized as providing a "band-aid" approach to health care, a critique that Justicia volunteers contend with in the previous chapter. Working with limited resources, many charity clinics can only provide the bare minimum in terms of primary care, including limited health screenings and access to medication. In discussing another local migrant health nonprofit, Cheryl described it as a place where patients could just get their prescriptions, saying, "It's kind of an assembly line of health care. Patients get in and get out with their scripts. There's not much more in terms of personalized care."

For CommUnity, these charity clinics would be examples of the "free versions of a broken system" against which they are defining themselves and their model of health care provision. As hinted in Cheryl's discussion, these clinics try to see as many people as they can each clinic day, resulting in less personalized care and more traditional patient-provider interactions. As an example, Grace in Action, another migrant health organization in Phoenix discussed in chapter 1, provides free health care to uninsured migrants but counts their number of patient *visits* each year, rather than the number of actual patients.[16] In contrast to this model of care, CommUnity emphasizes personalized care that takes into account not only the medical issues of each patient, but also the social, economic, and even psychological support that individual patients may need.

Although the volunteers at CommUnity certainly have reservations about the model of health care provided by these charity organizations, they remain diplomatic in their characterization of this medical provision, reserving their harshest critiques for the larger "broken system."

Instead, CCP characterizes the difference between their work and that of the charity clinics as one of quality versus quantity. As Michael described it,

> They are doing the work [of providing health care to uninsured migrants] too, and it's work that needs to be done. There's no way that we at CCP will ever be able to address the sheer demand for immigrant health care in Phoenix. So, we recognize the important work that they are doing. At the same time, we have chosen instead to emphasize quality over quantity.

For CommUnity, the privileging of quality care is much more than a strategic decision about the allocation of resources. This prioritization of quality care is integral to their alternative model of health provision that does not replicate the brokenness of the mainstream health system. In this way, CCP defines its work not only against the "broken systems" of immigration and health care but also in contrast with charity models of migrant health care in the US.

Clinic Vision: Immigrant Health Justice

CommUnity's emphasis on quality care is central to the clinic's alternate vision of "immigrant health justice." A medical student and CCP volunteer, Abeni, discussed CommUnity's work to create and model an alternative framework for migrant health care, saying, "What CCP is trying to do, rather than fight against the system all the time, which is just exhausting, they're like 'you know what, we're going to go over here and just build something new.'" More than a critique of migrant health care in the US, immigrant health justice asserts health provision for uninsured, undocumented migrants predicated on a rights-based approach to medical care. Immigrant health justice combines a recognition of health care as a human right with the strategic discursive framing of medical provision *as* activism.

In contrast to the exclusionary nature of the for-profit medical system, CommUnity asserts health care as a human right for everyone, but especially for undocumented and uninsured migrants. Donna, who is an outspoken advocate for universal health care, emphasized this value: "Health care is a fundamental, basic human right. I don't care how you got here or where you came from, every human has a right to health care." Beyond the right to health care, Adam, a board member and clinic volunteer who directs an international medical humanitarian organization, critiqued the hierarchy of health care quality and access in the US in an interview for a promotional film about the clinic's work: "Medical care is not a commodity that only a few should have because they have the right things in their pockets—money or papers. There cannot be a hierarchy of who gets health care and who doesn't . . . or who gets good health care and who has to just get what's left over. We should all get the same health care." For CommUnity, ensuring the right to health care for all is about more than access.

"Immigrant health justice" involves working toward a medical system in which undocumented and uninsured migrants in the US are able to access free health care that is not separate from or substandard to that which US citizens receive. Indeed, part of the clinic's formal mission statement defines immigrant health justice as the recognition of "the rights of all people to have accessible and equitable health services through an integrative, sustainable model." One of the fundraising appeals posted to the clinic's social media expounds on this vision:[17]

> We pride ourselves on being relentless in getting our patients what they need. Because of our network of literally hundreds of amazing volunteers . . . we're able to deliver high quality care to our patients for only about $200 per year per patient. That includes labs, home visits, and frequent appointments with a diverse and multidisciplinary team that includes MDs, PAs, RNs, Naturopathic doctors, acupuncturists, life coaches, case workers, physical therapists, and an amazing dedicated group of support staff ranging from phlebotomists to interpreters, and more. And the standard of care is far better than what a lot of wealthy people with good insurance get . . . you can help us give one of our immigrant neighbors the quality care and relentless follow-through that they need and deserve.

CommUnity characterizes the health care that it provides as accessible and equitable primarily because of the "relentless" nature of its "follow-through" and advocacy on behalf of its patients. The personalized care that patients receive through this "relentless follow-through" includes regular home visits for some of the clinic's most vulnerable patients, such as a young refugee father who was partially paralyzed after a stroke. Through multiple home visits a week, CCP volunteers provided material support in the form of food and childcare for his two young children, while others taught him how to walk again.

This accessibility of the CommUnity health care model includes recruiting volunteers who are native or fluent Spanish speakers and often migrants, who are currently or formerly undocumented themselves, so that CCP patients are met with volunteers who can communicate with them and empathize with their experiences. This attention to volunteers who share identity or experiences with the clinic's patients is echoed across many Third Net organizations, including Justicia y Paz, which also recruits native and fluent Spanish speakers as volunteers. From chapter 2, we see that Justicia residents (i.e., migrants) also often assume volunteer leadership opportunities within the organization and assist newer residents with navigating health care and social services. One of the Third Net's critiques of the mainstream health system focuses on the lack of language-appropriate and culturally competent care and specifically the lack of Spanish-speaking staff and interpreters that can communicate effectively with patients. This language barrier provides an additional—and largely unnecessary—barrier to care for patients who do not speak English fluently. CommUnity operates a large cadre of interpreters who are always present for the minority of volunteers who do not speak Spanish, and these non–Spanish-speaking volunteers are trained on the etiquette of using interpreters in their conversations with patients, including strict instructions to always speak directly to the patient themselves and not to the interpreters when discussing the patient's diagnosis and treatment plans.

Furthermore, CommUnity argues that the quality of care provided at the clinic is as good as, if not "far better than what a lot of wealthy people with good insurance get." For CCP, "quality" health care for their patients means providing the most comprehensive medical care possible within their capacity, and it is their definition of "quality" care that locates the work of the clinic in relation to both the mainstream formal health system and other Third Net organizations. On the one hand, this quality health care includes CommUnity's attempts to mirror the health services their patients would receive at a primary care clinic, if they had both health insurance and authorized immigration status. As will be discussed later in this chapter, these services are greatly constrained by the clinic's limited financial resources, the exorbitant cost of health services in the US, and the larger structural issues faced by their patients. In the absence of ability to provide comprehensive health care to its patients, the clinic has developed a patchwork of health services based on the specializations and expertise of the various volunteer health workers. This patchwork of care includes a range of health services from what we would consider typical Western medicine to holistic or alternative medicine. The fundraising appeal above lists a variety of health providers—from biomedical to naturopathic to holistic—that provide a comprehensive range of health "modalities" collaborating to meet patient needs. This holistic definition of health also encompasses a patient's mental and emotional well-being, providing trauma-informed care that addresses the distressing experiences of many of the clinic's patients prior to, during, and after migrating to the US as well as the chronic stress associated with living as undocumented in Arizona. Fundamental to CCP's migrant health justice work is a belief in what medical provision can accomplish for patients who have been systematically excluded, whose lives and health have been continually devalued. While the services CommUnity provides its patients try to replicate what insured patients access at a primary care clinic, part of its mission includes the *delivery* of these medical services in a manner that fosters dignity and respect for its patients, which low-income, uninsured, undocumented migrants often do not receive in the mainstream health system.

Building a Movement that Challenges the "Broken System"

As an alternate vision for migrant health care, migrant health justice frames health care provision *as* political advocacy, and in this way, CommUnity describes its work as "humanitarian activism" rather than charity. It is through migrant health justice that the clinic fulfills its mission of "not replicating a free version of a broken system." A social media post about the clinic's vision of immigrant health justice states,

> If you're a [CCP] supporter, you probably already know that we're more than just a regular clinic . . . We're not just prescribing pills—we're building

a movement and changing the culture of medicine in Phoenix. . . . In this time of increasingly hateful anti-immigrant rhetoric, it's one way to push back against the tide of hate, and make sure that immigrant and asylee families here in Arizona have the services they need and deserve—no matter what our politicians say about them. Together, we really can build a better world, where all our neighbors, regardless of immigration status, know that their lives and health are valued.

In this excerpt, migrant health justice as envisioned by CCP 1) challenges and counteracts hateful anti-immigrant rhetoric, 2) changes the dominant culture of medicine, and 3) builds a movement that spreads the vision and reality of immigrant health justice beyond the confines of the clinic.

Through the framework of immigrant health justice, CommUnity pushes back "against the tide of hate" and challenges anti-immigrant sentiment by framing migrants as *patients*. This assertion of the patient status of uninsured, undocumented migrants is the means through which CCP challenges the usual political rhetoric around migrants as social burdens or drains of collective resources. In addition, CCP uses its approach to health care provision as a means of "changing the culture of medicine in Phoenix." Indeed, part of the organization's vision statement is that "by challenging the dominant culture of healthcare, we seek to . . . inspire health justice advocacy." Changing the culture of medicine is ultimately a lofty goal, but CommUnity defines it first and foremost as being "more than just a regular clinic" that prioritizes far more than "just prescribing pills." In a documentary film about the clinic, Michael states emphatically,

> People will sometimes question our approach to care, especially our emphasis on home visits. They'll say, "Is that cost effective, because you just spent the entire day only seeing one or two patients?" No one ever asks if it's cost effective to let these people get sick and have them in the ICU. Nobody cares that it costs $60,000 for an ICU stay. That's just accepted. That's normal. We don't question it; we don't criticize it.

As Michael's critique demonstrates, the exclusivity and exorbitant costs associated with medical care in the formal system are more or less taken for granted, but the costs of *not* providing health care to unin-sured, undocumented migrants remain largely unquestioned. Shifting the responsibility of ill health from migrant patients to a larger struc-tural critique, CommUnity pushes back against the individualizing and patient-blaming narratives that vindicate or erase structural violence and the multiple oppressions experienced by uninsured, undocumented patients.

Finally, fundamental to CCP's characterization of its health provi-sion as more than charity care is the clinic's work to build a broader movement for immigrant health justice predicated on mutual solidar-ity. This vision seeks to realize "a better world, where all our neighbors, regardless of immigration status, know that their lives and health are valued." CommUnity volunteers recognize that this larger vision cannot be achieved as one community or clinic. Abeni hinted at this recogni-tion when she said, "One clinic can only make so much of a difference. We want to get the word out so that we can become a template for other clinics and work [that needs] to be done." Thus, through creating a clinic space where health care is provided not as charity but as part of a larger vision of immigrant health justice, CommUnity is working to create a model for other clinics and indeed the health care system as a whole, a model of what it can look like when health provision does not replicate the "brokenness of the system."

Part of this model includes eliminating a separation between health care for insured citizens and uninsured migrants. Indeed, clinic orga-nizers worked to deliver the same quality health care that they them-selves would want to receive. In fact, as our fieldwork at CommUnity was drawing to a close, one of the volunteer doctors at the clinic started a separate clinic day for people *with* insurance. This model was both symbolically and practically important for the clinic in challenging the charity model of care and for creating an alternative model of mutual solidarity. In effect, it was a testament to the quality of care at CCP that insured volunteers and community members would access the medical services at the clinic. It also provided a material benefit to CCP: the doc-tor charged his patients' insurance for their care and then donated this money to help run the clinic. In this way, insured patients directly con-tributed to the care for uninsured patients through a model of mutual solidarity. Not only does CCP argue that everyone should have access to the same quality health care regardless of socioeconomic or immigration status, but it also works to vision and create models of care within the current structural constraints of the US immigration and health systems that translate CCP's value of equitable, quality health care into practice.

Contestations over "Quality" Care

At its heart, migrant health justice is a radical approach to migrant health care that recognizes the structural failures of the immigration and health systems in the US and that asserts the right to quality health care for uninsured, undocumented migrants. Driven by a commitment to immigrant health justice, CommUnity volunteers work within the Third Net to make this radical vision a reality, in which their patients have a recognized right and access to free quality health care and they do not have to live in the shadows, in constant fear of being detained and deported away from their families and lives in the US. Working to achieve this vision in the midst of these "broken systems" creates some fundamental challenges for CCP, including having to deal with the structural constraints of immigration and health policy in Arizona and across the US and allocating their limited material resources to provide care for their patients.

These fundamental challenges that CCP faces in realizing its vision of immigrant health justice translate, in part, into organizational tensions and contestations over the definition and practice of "quality" health care for uninsured, undocumented migrants. As a result, two factions formed among clinic volunteers in contention over how to define and deliver "quality health care" in an equitable way. These two factions disagreed whether to privilege a "clinical" or "activist" approach. On the one hand, the "clinical" approach to migrant health justice asserts an understanding of quality care that aligns with achieving the health measures and standards of care. On the other hand, the "activist" approach invokes the clinic's history as "unapologetically activist" to argue that CommUnity's definition of quality should be based on working with the local migrant community to meet their most urgent health care needs while collectively mounting resistance to anti-immigrant measures in Phoenix. These factions of "clinical" and "activist" do not divide neatly along the type of health modality practiced by some of the volunteers.

For instance, volunteers who were biomedically trained health professionals and had day jobs in some aspect of the mainstream health system did not only adhere to the clinical faction; many were supportive of the activist vision that was more critical of broader notions and interpretations of "health." This divide within the clinic organizers ended up generally falling along the two different clinic days—with the organizers of the Thursday nursing clinic day more aligned with the activist faction and the Saturday clinic staff representing the clinical faction.

The activist faction was also seen as being more closely linked with the larger Phoenix migrant rights community, while the clinical faction was more closely linked with medical schools and other clinics and practitioners within the city. In considering these two perspectives at the clinic, Michael described their different approaches to health care provision:

> Organizations that are started by clinicians start off by saying, "How many resources do we have and what are we able to do with those resources? What's the best way to spend them?" Whereas an activist starts out by saying, "What needs to get done?" and then goes from there to "What do we have to do to make that possible?" It's a little bit of a different way of looking at the world. It's more seat of your pants and gutsy, and sometimes we're able to pull off things that didn't look possible.

In this quote, Michael describes the subtle but distinct differences in these two factions' approach. According to Michael, who identifies more in the activist faction, the clinical approach considers first and foremost the (very limited) resources available to the clinic and then works to equitably allocate these resources, which the volunteers with more activist leanings consider to be operating from a deficit model. Instead, they work to envision a reality in which migrants access free quality health care and then, taking patients' needs as their starting point, create collaborations and creative solutions to meet these needs as best as possible.

Although the tension between these two factions manifested in various ways within the clinic, the most contentious example is the patient waiting list. CommUnity faced a much larger demand for care from potential patients than it could accommodate. As a result, it maintained an ever-growing waiting list, which had been a point of contention at

CCP for years. Lack of transparency at the clinic raised questions from local Latinx and migrant communities about how patients on the waiting list accessed care at CommUnity. To dispel what clinic organizers interpreted as misinformation circulating in the community, CCP organizers created an advisory group of "members of the community," including mainly migrant and Latinx community leaders and friends of the volunteers. With the intent to ensure some community oversight of the clinic, this advisory group was tasked with putting together criteria for prioritizing which patients to take from the waiting list and in an order that would be deemed "fair." In addition to specific health needs, the criteria that the advisory board created also took into account social location in terms of a potential patient's family commitments and intersectional experiences of structural vulnerability.[18] For instance, a single mother with multiple children would be prioritized over an elderly man with no family.

According to some CommUnity organizers, mainly those in the "clinical" faction, the criteria that the group came back with was an "overly complicated" algorithm. As she recounted this episode in the history of the clinic, Donna said, "But then that meant that someone who had an A1C of nine[19] would sit on the waiting list, while someone who was prediabetic would get care. That just didn't make sense." Some organizers, like Donna, worried that this formula would mean that someone in imminent medical danger would languish on the waiting list without care, while someone with less urgent health needs would be allowed onto the clinic's roll. Instead of working with the advisory board to give different weight to aspects of the criteria in order to remedy these issues, these CommUnity organizers vetoed the advisory board's recommendations wholesale, declaring them to be too complicated. Thus, after creating the advisory board to cultivate more direct relationships and transparency with the local Latinx migrant community, upon receiving their recommendations, one faction of organizers within CCP's board ultimately disregarded the criteria. After this incident, the advisory board was effectively disbanded, which caused additional tension and strife between CommUnity and the wider Latinx migrant community in Phoenix.

To save face with this advisory board and the community, clinic organizers who had vetoed the criteria for prioritizing new patients had to skirt around the issue of the waiting list, instead creating a "simpler" system that they could use to attest to transparency and fairness. To balance these demands, the new policy dictated that they not take anyone off the waiting list until CCP had enough money in the bank (and enough volunteer capacity and room in the clinic) to cover the initial lab work and follow-up for *everyone* on the list. Meaning, when this financial solvency and organizational capacity is determined by the clinic's board, they will clear the entire waiting list all at once, accepting everyone on it as new patients. In this way, they attempted to bypass questions of transparency, fairness, and "overly complicated" determinations of deservingness. However, this "simpler" policy did not fix the damage done to the perception of the distance (and tension) between the clinic and the wider community. Unsurprisingly, the choice made by some of CommUnity's founding board members to ignore the criteria decided by the community advisory board irked the more activist-leaning CCP organizers.

Furthermore, the "simpler" system did not address the primary issue with the waiting list that drove the initial creation of the advisory board: people with severe chronic health conditions would still languish on the waiting list for months, if not years, until the clinic had enough resources and capacity to accept everyone on the list. To mitigate this issue, both factions of volunteers agreed on the need for a discretionary category of "emergency patient." These are patients whose conditions were acute enough to "skip" the considerable waiting list and be seen immediately. This designation mainly included people with severe and uncontrolled diabetes putting them at imminent risk for more serious health problems. In practice, the definition of "emergency" at CCP was ambiguous.

Emergency patients were accepted for new patient intake appointments at the Thursday clinic because it had more scheduling leeway than Saturdays, which were incredibly busy. Once the patient had their initial examination and their lab work results came back, they were scheduled for a follow-up visit on a Saturday to get any prescriptions and discuss their treatment plan. As a result of this arrangement, Thursday clinic organizers (who on the whole were more aligned with the "activist" approach to quality care) accepted more emergency patients. With his somewhat liberal interpretation of "emergency," Michael often faced pushback from Saturday clinic leaders for his seeming disregard of not only the established policies around taking new patients, but also the limited resources and financial strains the clinic faced in trying to deliver care to their existing patients. During the Saturday clinic, Ed would question the qualification of these new patients as "emergency" given the results of their lab work and would assume, sometimes rightly, that the Thursday organizers were using the emergency patient category as a loophole for accepting new patients. But other times, Ed would see only the objective health criteria of these new patients without taking into account the broader experiences of these patients that would qualify as "emergencies." Such a conflict arose around the emergency patient status that precipitated Juanita's acceptance as a patient. On paper, Juanita's lab work did not necessarily indicate that her diabetes was more uncontrolled or imminently dangerous than other patients waiting to be admitted to the clinic. But the numbers from her lab work did not capture the severe emotional trauma that she had endured nor the state of her mental health. Michael recounted a story to some of the clinic volunteers on the day of her initial appointment—Juanita and her children had witnessed the cartel torturing and murdering her husband and their father, which caused them to flee Mexico for the US. Her admission as an emergency patient led to a somewhat heated argument between Ed and Michael, the de facto leaders of the two factions at the clinic.

This argument between CCP organizers demonstrates the tensions that play out in terms of taking on new emergency patients. Because the clinical volunteers only examine the quantitative results from the vitals and bloodwork of new emergency patients, they miss many aspects of what constitutes these patients' emergencies. For instance, in the case of Juanita, her A1C levels demonstrated that she had type 2 diabetes but would not have indicated a more severe case of diabetes than other potential patients on the waiting list. This fact had spurred Ed's anger at Michael's perceived "overuse" of his discretion to accept emergency patients. However, the most important information about her health—the trauma she experienced from being forced to watch the cartel murder her husband and the mental health issues she faced as a result—did not appear in her bloodwork.

The waiting list is but one example of tensions within the clinic. However, this example does more than demonstrate some of the interpersonal conflicts at the clinic or the struggle to allocate inadequate resources to the clinic's patients. Rather, it illustrates the very real challenges and constraints in practice that the clinic organizers and volunteers experience when trying to achieve their radical vision of migrant health justice amid the current "broken systems" of immigration and health in the US.

Delivering a "Collage of Care"

In grappling with the structural constraints faced by their patients, many CommUnity organizers and volunteers conceive of health broadly—beyond lab results to include mental, emotional, and spiritual health—and combine a variety of approaches to health and well-being that enable the clinic to provide more services and treatments while challenging the structural violence experienced by their patients.[20] Because of the limited nature of the primary and specialist care available to undocumented migrants, the medical services offered by CommUnity incorporate a unique coexistence of various health approaches (or "modalities"), including biomedical, naturopathic, and holistic care. These modalities are focused on the prevention, where possible, and maintenance, where necessary, of chronic health conditions like diabetes that can quickly become costly, debilitating, and life-threatening in the absence of health care provision. This section examines the unique interrelationship between these various health approaches that are often in tension with one another but that coexist within the space of CCP, creating a "collage of care" for its patients that challenges the structural violence and medical racism[21] that patients encounter in the mainstream health system.

The concept of "continuum of care," which is central to theoretical and practical approaches to patient care and case management, refers to the "system that guides and tracks patients over time through a comprehensive array of health services spanning all levels and intensity of care."[22] This continuum of care involves a spectrum of social services and medical care—from preventative and wellness to primary and specialist to emergency and acute. However, this mainstream concept often assumes that the patient has access to health coverage and care as well as the financial means to pay for it. In the absence of eligibility for and access to comprehensive and integrated health care provision for its patients, Third Net clinics and providers must instead fashion what we call a "collage of care," which represents an ad hoc infrastructure of services from the limited resources available to low-income, uninsured, and undocumented patients. In the case of CommUnity, this collage of care involves the integration of various health modalities that are not usually found working together. In fact, they are often in direct tension with one another, as the supremacy of the biomedical model in health services in the US subsumes all others. A clinic space where Western biomedicine and other "alternative" health modalities coexist, CommUnity provides a collage of care predicated on the recognition of the multiplicities of precarity experienced by their patients, the limitations they face in terms of health care access and provision, and the legitimation of non-biomedical and non-Western health modalities.

The volunteers at CommUnity describe the various categories of health services they offer in their collage of care as 1) biomedicine, 2) "woo" medicine, and 3) "woo-woo" medicine. "Biomedicine" refers to clinical, allopathic, Western medicine that would be familiar to most people in the US who have health insurance and access to medical care. At CommUnity, the biomedical arm of the clinic is run by a team of volunteer doctors, nurses, physician assistants (PAs), PA students, and aspiring PA students trying to get volunteer experience in a clinical setting. This team of volunteers is able to provide limited primary care and some ad hoc specialist services, depending on what medical equipment was donated from local clinics and medical practices and what specific knowledge the volunteer medical professionals can share. For instance, the clinic has an EKG machine and volunteer technicians trained to read the machine's output, so CommUnity can provide EKGs, with no cost added to the clinic, to check for potential heart issues. However, if the EKG machine detects any abnormalities, the clinic struggles to find a place to refer the patient for specialist care. Like other Third Net organizations, CommUnity can only provide a patchwork of medical services in house and relies on the networks and knowledge of its volunteer medical professionals for referrals to the few primary care doctors and specialists who can provide pro bono or low-cost care as well as to time- and resource-constrained free health screening programs. In the absence of a more formal program that provides uninsured, undocumented migrants access to care in the mainstream system (e.g., Harris

Health's Gold Card described in chapter 2), this referral network is vital to CommUnity patients accessing specialist care.

"Woo" medicine corresponds to naturopathic and homeopathic health services involving herbs, vitamins, supplements, essential oils, acupuncture, and bodywork provided by a team of volunteer naturopathic doctors (NDs) and students. Naturopathic medicine works to "treat the whole person" physically, mentally, emotionally, environmentally, socially, and spiritually. Positioning itself against conventional allopathic medicine, naturopathic medicine uses the healing power of nature to address the underlying causes of illness, rather than treating the symptoms with prescription medications.[23] In the US, NDs can practice in only 19 states and the District of Columbia. Not only is Arizona one of these states, but the Phoenix area is home to one of seven naturopathic medical schools in the country. Although allopathic and naturopathic medicine have competing and somewhat contradictory philosophies, both MDs and NDs practice medicine together at CCP and consult with one another on many of the same patients.

"Woo-woo" medicine involves a range of holistic services performed by people with training in less conventional health modalities, from talk therapy to sound therapy to indigenous healing remedies provided by Spanish-speaking migrants from the community. One of the main volunteer holistic practitioners at CommUnity, Alondra, could be described as a curandera, a spiritual healer trained in a mixture of indigenous Aztec, Mayan, and Spanish shamanic and healing remedies. Alondra describes her work as "intuitive" coming from various apprenticeships with other curanderas, and she uses a variety of implements and techniques in her work, including feathers, rain sticks, didgeridoos, tuning forks, crystal singing bowls, and chanting. For some of CCP's patients, these healing remedies would be familiar from their home countries and more trusted than biomedicine. Another practitioner in the "woo-woo" camp, Octavia, practices hypnotherapy or talk therapy, although as a migrant she is unlicensed in the US. She will meet with patients who seem to be under considerable stress or struggling with their mental health and will talk through visualizations and mindfulness affirmations focused on helping the patient relax or cope with the everyday stressors they experience as undocumented, uninsured, low-income migrants struggling with chronic health issues. Alondra and Octavia regularly meet with patients after they have seen the biomedical or naturopathic volunteers, although the holistic practitioners' approach to health is most at odds with Western biomedicine.

Within the clinic setting at CCP, these three approaches to health compose an infrastructure or collage of care that focuses on prevention and maintenance of chronic health conditions. In the absence of a continuum of care and of patient eligibility for health insurance coverage, this combination of health approaches works together out of dire necessity, pooling resources and medical knowledge and overcoming disciplinary differences to provide whatever services they can for the patients' benefit. The majority of CCP's patients are on some part of the diabetic spectrum, which shows up in their initial blood work, and potentially their urinalysis, and other physical manifestations. Patients with blood levels that demonstrate they are "prediabetic"—at high risk for developing type 2 diabetes if measures are not taken to stall or reverse this course—are referred to both biomedical and naturopathic providers. In the absence of other health complications, the patient will be seen mostly by naturopathic practitioners, who through vitamins, supplements, nutrition education, and other interventions will work to keep the patient from developing diabetes. However, a patient who already has, or develops, diabetes will be seen almost exclusively by the allopathic providers, who will put the patient on an oral diabetes drug to attempt to further control their blood sugar and keep them from becoming insulin dependent. This treatment includes another level of education in which the patient is provided with a glucometer and taught to measure their blood sugar levels periodically throughout the day and then to record this information and share it with the provider.

A patient who is insulin dependent has already exhausted many of their options in terms of what the clinic has to offer and what they can access in the Third Net's collage of care. Insulin for uninsured diabetics is prohibitively expensive. Because generic versions are non-existent in the US, insulin can cost up to $500 per month, and the price has increased rapidly over the past several years. There are a handful of cheaper—and overall less effective—versions of insulin that are available at Walmart, which has a fairly comprehensive list of medications that it provides at a very low cost. However, the person using this less expensive insulin must be absolutely rigid about their diet and the particular times they take the insulin each day.

In the absence of access to health care and insurance, undocumented and uninsured migrants exhaust their health care options and become at-risk for acute health issues much earlier in the disease's trajectory than other diabetics. Thus, becoming insulin dependent is not just a nuisance that necessitates more expensive medical interventions but a life-threatening issue. Diabetes that has remained untreated and uncontrolled for years causes CommUnity patients serious health problems—from deteriorated eyesight, to neuropathy in the limbs that can lead to wounds that will not heal and eventually amputations, to kidney failure that requires regular dialysis (to which undocumented migrants do not have access). Additionally, undocumented diabetics with neuropathy who cannot access wound care may quickly lose limbs and, as a result, their ability to work. Clinic volunteers were particularly worried about a patient who worked in roofing but no longer had much feeling in his feet, making his job much more dangerous (similar to the person known to Justicia discussed in chapter 2). Furthermore, it is virtually impossible then for uninsured, undocumented diabetics facing kidney failure to get regular dialysis, much less a kidney transplant. Given the serious limitations of health care access for undocumented diabetic patients, the clinic focuses on the importance of preventative care and maintenance of chronic health conditions employing a variety of health modalities in a collage of care that may mean the difference between life and death for the patients. As such, multiple (and arguably contradictory) approaches to health care unite under the banner of "immigrant health justice" to provide health services to CCP's patients.

Conclusion

Through its mission and work, CommUnity challenges dichotomies of direct service provision and political advocacy, demonstrating the importance of health care advocacy in the face of intense migrant criminalization and revealing the inherent failings of immigration and health policy in the US. CCP's refusal to engage a charity model of migrant health care resists the conception of migrants as burdens in political discourse as well as the image of the deserving or suffering migrant that is central to Justicia's work (see chapter 2). This reframing of migrant health care turns the political rhetoric about migrant dependency on its head. Instead of providing charity care through a trickle-down model, it reframes migrant health care to involve the democratization of health care access and the redistribution of resources to address the structural inequalities associated with health and migration status in the US. As a result, CommUnity—and Third Net organizations like it—establishes migrant health care as political advocacy, framing health provision as a challenge to broader anti-immigrant rhetoric and the structural problems with for-profit health care and immigration enforcement. In this mission, CCP is seemingly successful at mobilizing discourses of migrants' patient status as a way to legitimate their work and critique systemic failures.

Through the discourse and practice of migrant health justice, CCP works toward both migrant rights and health justice. This migrant health justice approach, first and foremost, critiques 1) the for-profit health care system that excludes undocumented migrants from eligibility for health coverage and 2) punitive immigration policies and enforcement tactics that criminalize its patients. It also models migrant health care provision that works to disrupt discourses of deservingness and reveals the inherent structural issues with immigration and health systems in the US. In this way, CCP works to create broad social change and to build a movement of migrant health justice predicated on community solidarity.

As demonstrated in this chapter, the realities of translating this discourse into practice for organizations and clinics in the Third Net can be contentious. Although CommUnity volunteers are seemingly on the same page with supporting the mission of the clinic, the realities of delivering equitable quality health care in the Third Net force organizations to make difficult decisions about how to allocate care and resources and can lead to internal tensions. Although it may be easy to point to interpersonal conflicts as the sources of these tensions, it is important to instead be clear about the structural impossibilities that Third Net organizations face in providing care to their patients in the absence of their eligibility for health care in the mainstream system, their criminalization due to their immigration status, and the real barriers to free health care created by a larger privatized health system in the US. Similar to Justicia,

CommUnity Clinic's mission points to a discursive focus on the failures of this larger system, as well as a critique of other more charity-focused organizations that replicate these failures within the Third Net.

The following chapter analyzes yet another model of health care provision and migrant support in the Third Net through an organization called Houston Health Action (HHA). Predicated on a model of mutual aid, Houston Health Action demonstrates the power of community solidarity and peer support among a group of uninsured, undocumented migrants who have faced catastrophic injury and disability that puts them in need of acute, long-term health services.

4

Challenging Public Charge

The notion of migrants as "public charges" or burdens on society high-lights the contradictions in health care and immigration legislation and the embodied consequences of the intersecting oppressions of race, ability, immigration status, and health care access. In this chapter, we bring together disability and migration studies to understand how public charge, as an enduring administrative law and anti-immigrant ideology, functions to justify the exclusion of migrants from the formal health system, funneling them into the informal Third Net. In particular, we focus on a small nonprofit organization in Houston with an outsized vision of what community-based, mutual care can look like.

Houston Health Action (Health Action or HHA for short)[1] largely comprises Latinx, undocumented, and uninsured migrants who are survivors of catastrophic spinal cord injuries, stroke, or diabetes amputations. The executive director describes the members as "the people who have no meaning for the system."[2] They are trauma survivors who provide support for each other and educate others on how to manage the challenges that arise from navigating institutions and systems that perpetuate their exclusion.[3] Through this organization, we illustrate yet another model of how residents have responded to the virtually non-existent health care, particularly long-term care, for migrants. Their designation as public charges reinforces the characterization of them as unproductive and thereby disposable or deportable burdens. In response, Health Action members created their own sanctuary, or space of care, for themselves within the Third Net. They did so despite the fact that they do not have a health clinic, nor do any of the members have any biomedical expertise.

Unlike most mainstream health care organizations, Health Action does not accept a totalizing view of undocumented, low-income migrants as nothing but a social problem. Their stance is in line with a critical migration studies and a critical disabilities framework,[4] which uses an interdisciplinary analysis that combines the theoretical and method-ological tools of feminist/queer, ethnic, and transnational/postcolonial studies to de-center normative or dominant understandings of migrants and migration. Health Action's organizational infrastructure and mis-sion is explicitly created to 1) move away from a state-centric approach to migration that unquestioningly mimics the goals of national eco-nomic and political rationalities and 2) treat the experiences of migrants as more than victims or a problem to be solved (i.e., a suffering body). By centering the perspectives of the migrants themselves, Health Action provides important insights into not only this little-known sector of the Third Net, but also the larger health care system and the complex inter-sections of health and immigration policies.

Health Action members collectively organize within and against what they describe as an "apartheid" health care system.[5] Evoking a state-imposed system of racial segregation and discrimination, Health Action members are forthright in their direct challenge of the unequal immigration and health care system in the US and Texas. Their efforts to "decolonize the apartheid health system" incorporate a variety of tactics of care at multiple scales, including fundraising and organizing to obtain necessary medical equipment, providing emotional and moral support to each other to fight isolation, raising awareness and maintaining vis-ibility as undocumented migrants, and advocating for larger structural change and promoting intersectional social movements for individu-als with disabilities and people without health insurance or access to care. These actions are framed within a larger politics of decoloniza-tion, transforming their efforts as actions toward greater freedom from oppression through self-determination. Rather than a public burden, Health Action members are active global participants in an intersec-tional movement for greater justice and equality for everyone.

While the scope of our wider study informs the context and land-scape of the Third Net in which uninsured, low-income undocumented migrants operate, the case of Houston Health Action offers the perspec-tives and experiences of the only organization within our broader study to be led and operated by undocumented migrants. We met representa-tives of HHA in 2014 and again in 2015: first at a public meeting entitled "Health Care for All Texans," which called for support for a single-payer health system, and again at the organization's monthly meeting, where we met 27 Health Action members, all of whom are from Mexico and Central and South America. Building on the questions we asked of other individuals and organizations across our study sites and following the leads of participants, our interviews with Health Action members included discussions about the organization's leadership and activism within and beyond the local community, transnational relations with families in home countries, and health care for undocumented migrants in particular. The vantage points of HHA members vis-à-vis the Third Net offered critical analytical leverage that goes beyond describing post-ACA changes to the health care safety net and contributes idiosyncrasies from which to understand the health care system's infrastructure overall and its intersectional impacts of race, immigration status, and disability.

Building a Nation of Able-Bodied Migrants: Public Charge

In immigration law, public charge provisions allow for the exclusion of migrants from the US based on a largely discretionary determination of an individual's potential to become a public burden or "primarily dependent on the government for subsistence."[6] For over a century, public charge law has excluded migrants perceived to be or to have the *possibility of becoming* a burden on the state on both economic and medical grounds. It serves as the basis on which migrants are rendered inadmissible before and upon their arrival as well as illegal and deportable during their residence in the US.[7] It even allows for the forced removal or deportation of migrants who are documented as legal residents. Public charge operates as a sort of amorphous category that excludes migrants at the discretion of immigration officials. As a foundation of immigration law, public charge governs who is admissible to the country and thus has been central to the US colonial, nation-building project, determining which migrants are desirable and deserving of inclusion.

In its early stage, during the mass migration of Europeans during the turn of the last century (1892–1920), public charge was the most frequently used category of exclusion. According to historian Martha Gardner, "Between 1880 and 1924, 'likely to become public charge' provided a catch-all category of exclusion through which vast numbers of immigrants found themselves deported as potential paupers for moral, marital, physical, and economic deficiencies."[8] Immigration legislation during this time established that potential migrants could be excluded from admission to the US or deported for up to five years after their arrival for becoming a public charge for medical or economic reasons.[9] Subsequent immigration and welfare legislation since the 1950s has reaffirmed the government's powers of exclusion and expulsion on the basis of public charge and asserted that the use of public assistance demonstrates the public charge status of a migrant.[10] As such, public charge has played a fundamental role in the creation of the US citizenry as a nation of immigrants, directly defining the quality and character of those immigrants who are worthy of inclusion.

In addition, Douglas Baynton notes the centrality of normative understandings of ability and disability in the administrative implementation of public charge. He argues, "A disability analysis is essential . . . to making sense of the depth of anti-immigrant sentiment and the workings of immigration policy at the turn of the twentieth century."[11] Since this administrative law operates ideologically to produce and maintain the boundaries of deservingness and citizenship for migrants, it has privileged able-bodied migrants as potential productive citizens. Consequently, it has helped define the desirable migrant as a "good industrial citizen: one who would remain healthy, be a useful worker, and not become dependent on the charity of the nation,"[12] in contrast to those who are unproductive, non-contributing burdens or drains on the state.

Linked with these notions of deservingness are implicit and explicit characterizations of "good" migrants as productive and able-bodied, in contrast with public charges as disabled and dependent. In addition, by allowing migrants to be removed after living in the US for a number of years, public charge renders migrants deportable when they become "unproductive" for medical or economic reasons. This includes migrants who develop a disability as a result of an accident or long-term illness as well as those who are no longer able to work due to their age or the toll of years of manual labor on their bodies.

More than a century later, public charge remains a powerful tool in its strategic ambiguity. It is a statutory provision under the jurisdiction of nonjudicial staff and not subject to oversight by legislatures or courts. While other administrative laws evolved during the 20th century, public charge determinations remained in a stage of arrested development as it moved out of public view. Since the height of its application in the 1920s to the 1990s, public charge determinations were limited largely to the confines of American consulates abroad.[13] There, many potential migrants are denied visas by American consular officials for their likelihood of becoming a public charge without ever setting foot in the US.

The US Citizenship and Immigration Service (USCIS) refined the definition of "public charge" for the first time in 1999, after considerable pressure from legal advocates to clarify the ambiguous nature of this law. The one-page notice of clarification included this statement: "'public charge' means an individual who is likely to become primarily dependent on the government for subsistence, as demonstrated by either the receipt of public cash assistance for income maintenance or institutionalization for *long-term care* at government expense."[14] While the 1999 clarification allayed fears regarding the potential reach of public charge law for some, migrants who receive cash assistance and/or long-term care were specifically identified as socially burdensome, heightening their status as deportable.[15]

This clarification came about after several lawsuits successfully challenged how this administrative law was used in a Medicaid fraud detection program targeting migrants in California. Riding on the wave of anti-immigrant sentiment in 1994 that successfully propelled California's Proposition 187—a ballot measure that was subsequently deemed unconstitutional in severely limiting access to public benefits for undocumented migrants—the California Department of Health Services and the federal immigration authorities coordinated to force *documented* migrant women who legitimately used public health insurance (Medi-Cal) for prenatal care and delivery to repay the cost of their health care by designating them a public charge. In a study of this program, researchers found that low-income Latina and Asian migrant women traveling outside the country were stopped, fined, and even refused reentry to the US as a potential public charge at ports of entry, including the border of California and Mexico, the San Francisco International Airport, and the Los Angeles International Airport for legally using health insurance during the previous five years.[16] This fraud detection program was in existence for five years until it was terminated in 1999, after a damning state audit found the programs "poorly administered, inadequately planned, and legally liable" for overstepping the scope of their authority because they had attempted to influence federal immigration decisions on whether to admit or deport migrants and improperly shared confidential medical information in the process.[17] Once the program modified its operation in accordance with the required rules and protections, it no longer produced a favorable return on their investment. In fact, the cost of running the program exceeded the return.

As short-lived as it was, the California fraud detection program was devastating for thousands of low-income California residents and their families who had to pay thousands of dollars that they could not afford or who were denied reentry to the US. It was also an embarrassing failure for the government agencies involved as it became clear that the program was caught manufacturing "fraud" where it did not exist. The real fraudulent actor in this scheme was the government.

More recently, immediately following Donald Trump's presidential inauguration, his administration focused on public charge in their attack on migrants. They began by withdrawing the 1999 clarification and significantly expanding the definition of who is a public charge.[18] In a series of internal memos dating from 2016, the Department of Homeland Security proposed new guidelines to greatly expand those considered "inadmissible" for using or appearing *likely to use* public benefits, for which they are eligible.[19] Categories of affected public benefits included Supplemental Security Income (SSI), Supplemental Nutrition Assistance Program (SNAP, formerly the Food Stamp Program), and Children's Health Insurance Program (CHIP).

These restrictions targeted those applying for admission to the US as well as those already here applying for adjustment of their temporary immigration status to lawful permanent resident. More insidiously, it kept migrants, regardless of their legal status, from using public benefits for which they are eligible. This change eliminated significant avenues to migrate legally as well as remain in the US legally, and consequently created greater pressure for "illegal" methods of entry. Also of concern were the administrative procedures used to make a public charge determination. Information was gathered from a wide range of federal agencies, including the Internal Revenue Service, the Social Security Administration, and the US Department of Health and Human Services, as well as the applicant's personal medical records.

Certainly, retroactively punishing documented migrants who use public benefits for which they are eligible raises serious legal and procedural issues. But more important are the constitutional, political, and moral concerns resulting in public charge determinations and subsequent punishments of all migrants—documented or not. This federal effort by the Trump administration was based on the erroneous assumption that "households headed by aliens (legal and illegal) are much more likely than households headed by native-born citizens to use federal means-tested public benefits."[20] This is untrue. In fact, studies show that low-income migrants actually use less welfare than low-income native-born populations. Leighton Ku and Brian Bruen's 2013 study is just one among many that have found that migrants use less public benefits, including Medicaid, SNAP, cash assistance, and SSI.[21]

This effort also highlights the disingenuous rhetoric of anti-immigrant groups that call for harsh measures against "illegal" or "bad" migrants because it harms the "legal" or "good" migrants. This rhetoric softens the racist implications of anti-immigration efforts by alluding to purported "good" migrants. In actuality, there is no difference. In fact, "illegal migration" measures are simply a foil for the real target of all migrants. This was evident in the Trump administration's shift in allowing public charge law to exclude not only those who become entirely destitute and dependent on the government but potentially *every* migrant who *might* use some government-funded benefits.

The election of President Joe Biden in 2020 brought public charge policies back to the 1999 "field guidance," putting the legitimate use of health, nutrition, and housing programs by migrants outside the purview of public charge determinations once again.[22] As of this writing, the Trump-era rules are no longer in effect but the volatility of this potentially far-reaching federal policy from one presidential administration to another is unsettling. The earlier attempt in California to punish migrants for receiving benefits to which they are legally entitled should have given us pause before initiating such draconian policies. Instead, where California stopped its public charge expansion, the federal government took over, to far greater effect. Another potential lesson from California is that it was these kinds of extreme laws that undermined the legitimacy of the governmental agencies involved and created the turning point for the state's growing Latinx and Asian electorate and the rise of Democrats. But, more than 20 years later, extreme federal politics and policies targeting low-income migrants continue unabated. For instance, since COVID-19 began, research has documented that migrants are avoiding critical health and economic support due to public charge concerns. The Urban Institute conducted a survey of community-based organizations and found nearly 70% reported that public charge and other anti-immigrant policies deterred migrants from seeking COVID-19 testing and treatment, for which they are eligible.[23]

It is evident that while specific federal public charge policy clearly has significant impact on the health and well-being of migrants, it is also the case that a broader set of beliefs that presumes migrants to be a public burden has a pervasive effect in migrants' everyday lives.

Migrant Deservingness and the Fraying Safety Net in Texas

Given the strong public perception that migrants in general—even those deemed exceptional or "good"—are undeserving of health care due to their non-citizen status, migrants with disabilities, without insurance coverage or legal documents, and in need of long-term care are particularly vulnerable. A safety net health care administrator in Houston succinctly described the long-term care options for uninsured patients as "very little and very limited." She added, "we do our best with what we have. But that's difficult. It's hard to place someone when there's very little places to go."[24]

As a result of its refusal to expand Medicaid and to implement a state health insurance exchange, Texas is a unique site for the study of ACA implementation and the current state of the Third Net, as we have already discussed in previous chapters. Within Texas, Harris County presents a paradoxical case for migrant health care: it boasts a world-renowned medical infrastructure for state-of-the-art health care and, at the same time, it is home to the highest population of uninsured people in the country, a significant proportion of whom are migrants.

Within this great medical divide, Houston Health Action demonstrates the acute and intersectional marginalization experienced by uninsured and undocumented migrants with disabilities in the US at the point at which the expansion of health care coverage (through the ACA) is most dramatic in recent history. A nonprofit, independent organization, HHA was founded in 2005 by low-income migrant residents with spinal cord injuries who lacked access to health care and other social services. Most of the organization's members are Latinx, undocumented, and uninsured and are largely unable to maintain employment due to their injuries. HHA formed when Harris Health System no longer covered necessary medical equipment, primarily catheters, which for paraplegics who rely on wheelchairs for mobility are vital to their daily health needs.

In comparison to the formal Harris Health safety net system, Houston Health Action is minuscule. The organization does not appear on any list of safety net health care services, and yet, it is a lifeline for its members. Tomás, a board member of Health Action, succinctly explained in an interview (in Spanish), "Thank god we have [HHA], but living day to day is very difficult."[25] The organization employs one paid half-time staff person and has assisted hundreds of migrants with spinal cord injuries.[26] The 50 members of the organization are dedicated volunteers who meet three times every month to discuss what medical supplies and medications are needed or available, to plan fundraising efforts for these supplies, and to coordinate advocacy efforts to share information with the larger community. HHA's executive director, Diego, explained,

> We formed after Harris [Health System] denied our care and would not cover basic necessities like catheters, diapers, etc. We began by selling flowers by the side of the street to raise funds. Now, our group provides and distributes catheters [and other medical equipment], fundraise, and organize communities to get the word out about what is happening. Now, even citizens who are insured but can't afford these basic necessities are coming to us.[27]

Diego's statement touches on the long-term care struggles for people with disabilities in Texas. As Harris Health privileges the enrollment of those eligible for the ACA federal health insurance, individuals who still cannot afford health care or are undocumented and ineligible for coverage are left to fend for themselves. Health Action is a collective response to this void and, in times of crisis, extends its assistance to the larger community. In a self-published report documenting the devastating impact of Hurricane Harvey in August 2017 on its members, HHA stated,

It is ironic that, in these times when a cynical administration pushes anti-immigrant policies one after another—including mean spirited changes to the "public charge" rules aimed against the poor, the elderly and those with a disability—a group formed by immigrants with disabilities is proudly supporting citizens and non-citizens, not because we want to make a point, but because we recognize our shared human dignity.[28]

Health Action members understand intimately what it means to live within the paradox of being uninsured in a region replete with medical resources. They pointedly note that migrant communities, people with disabilities, people of color, and low-wage workers were already living in "policy created disaster zones,"[29] enduring years of defunding, privatization of public services, and racial criminalization in Texas before the onset of hurricanes and pandemics. They write, "We have seen people living in terrible conditions not due to a lack of resources in our society, but due to the callous insensitivity of those in power at the federal and state level and the pervasive inequality in access to resources and opportunities."[30]

Such callousness is particularly apparent in the lack of long-term care options. Long-term care encompasses a broad range of services and support over a prolonged period of time for those with chronic injuries or disabilities. The purpose of this kind of care is to minimize, rehabilitate, or compensate for loss of independent physical and mental health.[31] Typically, long-term care is categorized into two areas: 1) activities of daily living (ADL) such as bathing, dressing, using the toilet, and other personal care, and 2) instrumental activities of daily living (IADL) such as household chores, life management, medication management, and transportation. Most services in long-term care are generally low-tech, although some recovering from an acute, recent medical condition may need more medically oriented care such as intravenous therapy, wound care, and ventilator assistance.[32] The goal of long-term care is to create a good quality of life for those with disabilities by addressing their basic clinical and functional needs.

Although Health Action works to address its members' health needs as best it can, Diego acknowledges the limited ability to meet these needs in the absence of health care coverage for its members. In our interview, Diego said, "We provide both service and community organizing. The current system is not sustainable. We're all volunteers and we need to do so much more. We need to grow and fundraise."[33] Health Action members report increasing barriers to emergency care after the implementation of the ACA, and Diego said that wait times worsened, as did the quality of medical care in emergency rooms and community clinics. For Health Action members, their disability coupled with their immigration status make them easy targets for exclusion. HHA members' interactions with the formal safety net system (i.e., the Harris Health System) are a constant reminder of this vulnerability. Within the current system, policies require that their medical condition be "emergencies" before they can be treated. In this way, these emergencies and subsequent construction of undocumented migrants as public charges are manufactured by the health care system itself.

Jose's experience offers an example of this phenomenon. Jose, a Health Action member, was gravely injured in 1998 when he was struck by a car while biking to work in Houston. The drunk driver who hit him fled the scene and was never identified. As a result, Jose is paraplegic and relies on a wheelchair for mobility. He explained that one of the most profound and basic changes to his everyday life after his injury is the necessity of urinary catheters. He generally needs 200 catheters a month, but the cost is prohibitive, as he has little to no income. Without an adequate supply, he is forced to wash and reuse the normally disposable single-use catheters repeatedly, putting him at risk for catheter-associated urinary tract infections (CAUTI).

Although they are relatively simple plastic tubes, catheters are vital to the daily health and well-being of Health Action members, and a lack of access to an adequate supply of sterile catheters means that they suffer from repeat infections. Denying access to catheters is counterintuitive for those concerned about health care costs. Although it is one of the most common health care–associated infections in the US, CAUTI can be easily prevented through the use of sterile catheters. Compared to the costs of catheters (less than $1 each), medical treatment for CAUTI is astronomical, with each incidence of infection costing thousands of dollars to treat in a hospital.[34] When treated under emergency conditions, these costs rise sharply.

For Jose and others, dealing with infections is a protracted ordeal. As an undocumented migrant ineligible for health care coverage, Jose has to be near death for his condition to be warranted an "emergency" to access care in the emergency room. At one point, when Jose visited two different area hospitals, his urinary tract infection was not considered serious enough to be an emergency, and he was turned away. Due to his chronic health issues associated with his injury, Jose finds even the journey to and from the hospital to be excruciatingly painful. Later, when this infection spread to his other organs and he became gravely ill, he was taken by ambulance to the same emergency room that had earlier turned him away, deemed ill enough to receive emergency medical care, and finally given some medical attention for his infection. However, due to his status as an uninsured migrant, he was released from the hospital without necessary medication, which he could not afford to purchase out of pocket.

Another Health Action member, Samuel, described a similar set of events. Samuel's persistent catheter-associated urinary tract infections and lack of access to care took a toll on his body, resulting in kidney failure. Samuel now requires regular dialysis yet is deemed ineligible for dialysis except as an emergency. This means that, in order to get dialysis for his kidney failure that resulted from an untreated CAUTI, Samuel has to wait until his potassium level reaches a critical point before a hospital will treat him, placing him at risk of coma or death.

In describing the interaction of Health Action members with the formal health system, Diego stated, "'Good health' is defined in such a way that those whose bodies do not conform are not respected. So you get used to living with pain. It's the new normal."[35] This bodily nonconformity intersects in a number of ways to produce the marginalization that they endure as uninsured, undocumented Latinx migrants with disabilities. Their struggle with lack of access to health care and medical supplies represents the material consequences of the ideology of public charge that stigmatizes them as dependent, unproductive, and undeserving. Health Action's critique of this system is to denaturalize what Diego describes as "the new normal" by emphasizing the injustice of the current health system and by arguing for health care as a public good and health care access as a social justice issue. Diego says, "We don't have immigration reform. We don't have health care reform. We have apartheid. This is an apartheid system."[36]

Most Houston Health Action members and those they serve were injured in accidents on the job, while others were victims of crime, like one member we interviewed who was shot during a robbery and sustained kidney and spinal damage. Nationally, low-income undocumented migrants work in some of the most dangerous workplaces. In Texas, construction workers are 4.5 times as likely to be killed on the job as the average worker, making construction work the most dangerous occupation.[37] After farming and agricultural work, construction is the second-most-prevalent area of work for undocumented migrants,[38] and a number of Health Action members sustained catastrophic injuries while working on construction sites.

Christine Kovic argues that these workplace "accidents" suffered by undocumented migrants are not random. "These are more than mere 'accidents;' they point to the unequal and structural violence disproportionately experienced by members of marginalized communities. . . . Workplace injuries, like human rights abuses, are not equally distributed; some bodies are more vulnerable to injury than others."[39] HHA members experience this structural violence along multiple axes. Compounding the disproportionately high numbers of domestic and foreign-born racial/ethnic minorities in employment sectors with higher rates of workplace injuries,[40] the health care system sustains, rather than remedies, the injuries of undocumented migrants. They are denied care on the basis of their legal status, until their bodies are rendered medical emergencies, thus fulfilling the narrative of migrants as public burdens. The current system of care does not allow for prevention. Rather, migrants are required to be in a clear state of crisis, on the brink of death, to be "saved."

At the same time, the lack of long-term care options for undocumented and low-income migrants is used by hospitals to justify their attempts to unload or "dump" their patients to other Third Net organizations or even other countries. This is a refrain relayed repeatedly by hospitals, journalists, attorneys, and policymakers struggling to address the severe barriers to health care access for migrants. For instance, a 2011 story in the *Houston Chronicle* outlined how the University of Texas Medical Branch at Galveston (UTMB) attempted to forcibly repatriate (i.e., deport) Francisco Martinez to Mexico when they could not find a long-term care facility to take him. According to the reporter,

Still, the real problem isn't hospitals, which transfer most all patients, both U.S. patients and illegal immigrants, once urgent care is no longer needed and the bed is needed for other patients. It's long-term care facilities, unable to afford to accept patients, like Martinez, who don't have insurance. It remains for hospitals, obligated by federal regulation to arrange post-hospital care for those who need it, to find alternatives and to provide care indefinitely if they can't.[41]

This is a sympathetic recounting of hospitals "stuck" with few options. The impact for Francisco Martinez, however, is graver. Martinez, 37, broke his back on August 17, 2011, when he fell off a ladder while working on the roof of a bait shop. He became paralyzed from the chest down and had limited use of his hands.[42] His employer did not provide any benefits including worker's compensation or health insurance, and given his undocumented status, he is ineligible for Medicaid. After medically stabilizing Martinez, UTMB offered him a ticket to Mexico and repeatedly pressured him to sign a document stating that he voluntarily wants to leave the country. Martinez refused. He did not want to leave his wife, who is a US citizen, and their six-month-old child.[43] He recalls telling the hospital social worker, "if you don't want me here, just throw me outside."[44]

An estimated 12 million people, or 4% of the total population of the US, rely on some form of long-term care.[45] What might be surprising to many is that only a slight majority of the entire long-term care population is elderly. So, while the proportion of the population needing long-term care does rise with age, those younger than 65 are almost as large a group. However, the vast majority—in fact, four-fifths—of national long-term care spending is devoted to the elderly; and much of these funds are spent on institutional services or nursing homes.[46] In actuality, most long-term care is informal, unpaid, and provided by family, partners, friends, and neighbors in a person's home.[47]

The overall long-term care system in the US is threadbare and rife with problems. It does not come close to meeting the existing needs, puts catastrophic emotional and financial burdens on individuals and their families, and exists within a persistent bureaucratic tangle in which state and federal governments disavow their responsibility in funding and administering this crucial service.[48] One-fifth of adults with long-term care needs who live in the community (meaning, outside of nursing homes) report an inability to get the care they need, often with serious consequences.[49] In addition, despite reforms of nursing home regulation over the last few decades, reports indicate about a quarter of more than 17,000 nursing homes nationwide continue to have serious deficiencies.[50]

In comparison, health care for uninsured, undocumented migrants is even more threadbare, and long-term care for this population is virtually nonexistent. Without health care coverage, most Health Action members are completely dependent on care provided by family members. However, some members do not have family living in the Houston area or elsewhere in the US, and others have been left without care when their family members were deported. As such, immigration policy regarding deportation and removal has a significant impact on the health care of these individuals as well as on the health care costs in caring for this population. Consequently, for Health Action members, the loss of family is devastating in profound ways.

The few members who do not have family are forced to live in "personal care homes" or shelters (as discussed earlier in chapter 2). This option is viewed as the last resort, given the seemingly random and wide variation in quality of care. Health Action members have witnessed the conditions of these homes over the years during their regular visits with fellow members. "You can't imagine how bad some of these places are," Raul said (in Spanish). "They are not given proper care. And they are next to other people with severe mental and physical injuries in a tiny room. There is no rest."[51] Raul explained that this is what happens when health care resources and family care networks are absent. HHA has supported these members by visiting them and checking in on their care to ensure that their basic needs are met.

Health Action's destigmatization efforts occur on both the personal and structural levels. In addition to providing necessary medical supplies and participating in social movement organizing around migrant, labor, and disability rights, Houston Health Action combats the isolation their members experience on a personal level by providing the moral and emotional support that is vital for their community. Jose explained that members visit each other in hospitals, nursing homes, or personal care homes, wherever they are. "It's about the back and forth, the laughter, and good conversation [they provide each other]," he said.[52] Diego added, "We're trying to create community, a sense of belonging, for our well-being."

Intersecting Disabilities, Mutual Aid, and Long-Term Care

When we asked HHA members what they liked about Houston, almost all respondents initially responded with surprised silence. One member broke the silence with "Nada" (nothing). We then asked, "Why do you stay?" Each member replied, "Familia." Others added, "Houston Health Action." As part of their project of challenging the current hierarchical, unjust health care system, Health Action re-envisions the family as a community of care that transcends biological relationships. They also reimagine the traditional relationship of care, where someone who is able-bodied looks after someone with a disability, challenging it by articulating the ways in which they care for each other. They counter notions of public charge, which deems them "unproductive burdens"[53] on society. In fact, the group is writing a do-it-yourself health care handbook of advice and information for other undocumented and uninsured people with recent spinal cord injuries, discussing topics like where to get care, how to avoid infection, how to take care of scars, and where to find attorneys for those who have been in accidents. Through Health Action, these migrants collectively care for each other and pass along their hard-earned knowledge of how to provide mutual aid for everyone. For instance, in 2018, the group distributed $110,000 in medical supplies and $28,000 in medical equipment and now, area hospitals and social service agencies regularly refer the uninsured and underinsured—both US citizens and undocumented residents—to HHA.[54] It is apparent that the Third Net provides important support for the formal safety net in Houston.

The act of ordinary people responding to community needs and sharing resources, in conjunction with social movements demanding transformative change, is the definition of mutual aid.[55] Dean Spade writes, "At its best, mutual aid actually produces new ways of living where people get to create systems of care and generosity that address harm and foster well-being."[56] And while moments of spectacular crisis highlight the necessity of mutual aid, this mode of survival—of meeting people's needs and mobilizing collective resistance—is a persistent strategy adapted by many groups across the world. It is notable that COVID-19 brought awareness of the value of masking and ventilation in ways that those with certain forms of chronic illnesses and disabilities have experienced for years. Mel Chen writes, "we see how slowly a habitus can be learned; many of my excellently trained colleagues who wield magnificently expansive frameworks for thinking about matter seem remarkably unprepared and reactive to managing their air differently under these conditions."[57] For Health Action, then, every day is an emergency and their accumulated knowledge is valuable for the broader society. Rather than a public burden, they are a public resource.

Houston Health Action draws on multiple social movements—migrant rights, disability rights, and health care—to challenge the structures and policies that intersect to render undocumented migrants and people with disabilities invisible. As their central organizing strategy, the members of HHA address the increasing marginalization of migrant health care access by making themselves visible. Despite the difficulty and pain of mobility and vulnerability of their immigration status, Health Action members have made their visibility central in their efforts toward social change. As such, they have been integral to the migrant rights movement in Houston and across Texas. "Let's face it," Diego explained. "The way things work benefits some people. We need large numbers. We have to frame this as a community issue, beyond an individual issue."[58]

Health Action members regularly participate in, and even lead, migrant rights marches in Houston, representing their demands for greater worker rights, human dignity, and social equality. They place their bodies and their wheelchairs in front of media cameras, visually encompassing the collective action moving through the streets. At the same time, HHA acknowledges the difficulty of working within the "intersection" of migrant rights and health care access movements. According to Diego, given the range of complex issues surrounding low-income migrants, usually a singular concern that seems the most urgent receives all the attention and energy. The members make decisions regarding what actions to take based on how they might politically articulate their own intersectional experiences and identities. One member explained, "We need long-term campaigns with education about immigrants and health care. We have to keep fighting."[59] In addition to migrant rights marches and educational campaigns, Health Action members have also traveled to Austin and to Washington, DC, to lobby for disability rights, and they have tried to meet with the governor of Texas, Greg Abbott, who is himself paraplegic and uses a wheelchair for mobility.

Overall, Health Action's strategies intentionally stretch our understanding of health care to make a broader, infrastructural claim. Their efforts resemble what Deva Woodly calls "structural care," in which the purpose of care is to heal social ills as much as it is to heal individual wounds, and interdependence is affirmed as a necessity to do so.[60] Miriam Ticktin writes that such stances are part of a larger history of radical collective care, one that anti-racist activists and transnational feminists have articulated as based upon mutual social relations, not predicated on a show of deservingness.[61] At the same time, disability movement activists have worked to develop a "social" model of disability, rather than medical. Like other movements for social change, those working for disability rights identify systems of oppression as the problem and move away from medicalizing individual bodies as the problem. According to disability activist Eli Clare, it is ableism that needs a cure.[62]

In fact, in 1975, a British-based network of people with disabilities formed the Union of the Physically Impaired Against Segregation (UPIAS) to reject liberal and reformist campaigns of more mainstream organizations and argue for opportunities to participate fully in society—"to live independently, to undertake productive work and to have full control over their own lives."[63] As part of the UPIAS's Fundamental Principles of Disability statement, they wrote, "In our view, it is society which disables physically impaired people. Disability is something imposed on top of our impairments, by the way we are unnecessarily isolated and excluded from full participation in society. Disabled people are therefore an oppressed group in society."[64]

In distinguishing disability (social exclusion/oppression) from impairment (physical limitation), the latter is individual, private, and medical and the former is structural, public, and social.[65] Accordingly, the fight for disability rights is a fight for civil rights, and charity and pity actually contribute to exclusion and oppression. However, this particular framing of disability also has its own limitations. Others within activist and scholarly communities with disabilities have expressed concern about how impairment is understood, including understanding impairment as so clearly distinct from the social and structural, and the equation of disability with oppression so that one's identity as a disabled person is synonymous with oppression. The question, then, is never whether people with disability are oppressed in a particular situation, but rather, only the extent to which they are oppressed.[66] At the same time, activists have stressed the importance of acknowledging experiences of impairment that are a significant part of everyday life for those with disabilities.[67] Feminist philosopher Susan Wendell argues that it is possible to both understand disability as a social condition and take seriously impairment beyond medical norms of individual body and mind.[68] While the medicalization of disability, in which disability is regarded solely as individual misfortune and people with disabilities as suffering primarily from physical and/or mental abnormalities that only medicine can treat, cure, or prevent has been detrimental to conceptualizing the larger social construction of this social problem, Wendell points to the particular realities of illness and impairment that need to be addressed within conditions of "unhealthy" disability.

Houston Health Action presents just such a model. Its strategies illustrate how an organization can interweave their various intersecting conditions or oppressions to identify the larger social problems while addressing their immediate illness and pain. However, it is also the case that Health Action is faced with severe limitations due to these same oppressions and their intersecting impacts. Fundamentally, the point of long-term care is to ensure the opportunity for full political participation and social engagement rather than narrowly fixating on specific illnesses that are restricted to the expertise of medical professionals and administrators. Clearly, there is strong opposition to this vision of long-term care and such active political engagement by low-income migrants of color.

For years, people have been waiting for a seismic change in long-term care once baby boomers began to feel the pressure of caring for their parents.[69] This did not happen. These two generations did not join together as predicted to create a political movement to fix what everyone agrees is a broken system. Instead, the mentality of individual responsibility that helped pass the 1996 federal Personal Responsibility and Work Opportunity Reconciliation Act, known as welfare reform, works to keep the system as it is. Joshua Weiner writes, "When baby boomers discuss the difficulties of coping with the long-term care needs of their parents, they almost always see their trials as only a personal rite of passage, instead of a sign of systemic problems in need of repair. Until the personal becomes political and politics drives policy, it seems unlikely that much will change."[70]

There is continued concern that any initiative to "fix" the long-term care system may open access to those deemed undeserving by earlier welfare and health care reform efforts, in particular low-income migrants who were explicitly targeted for exclusion. Any efforts to improve home- and community-based services that increase costs, even initially, are abandoned.[71] This is despite evidence that these programs are successful in significantly increasing satisfaction among both patients/clients and caregivers.

And, as extensive as the Affordable Care Act was, it did not change the state of long-term care at all. In fact, what little was initially proposed was later deemed unfeasible by the Obama administration. The proposed Community Living Assistance Services and Supports, or CLASS Act, was intended to create a public, voluntary insurance program to help those with "mild" disabilities to remain living at home or in the community rather than having to move into a nursing home. The provision was supposed to be self-sustaining, with premiums for low-income and student enrollees at an extremely low level, which would require all others to pay more for their coverage. In a letter to Congress, then Secretary of Health and Human Services Kathleen Sebelius explained that it was impossible to devise a long-term benefit plan that would be "both actuarially sound for the next 75 years and consistent with the statutory requirements."[72]

As of now, long-term care for those with disabilities and chronic illnesses remain inadequate, uncoordinated, confusing, and underfunded. And families across the US provide much of the care needed to the detriment of their own health and financial security. Current political conditions would rather keep the "broken" system as is than allow migrants and other marginalized populations to access it.

Conclusion

Legal scholar Lori Nessel writes, "Throughout the world, migrant workers perform the most hazardous work for the lowest wages. However, when migrant workers or their family members are injured or become seriously ill and require ongoing medical treatment, they find themselves at the intersection of two unforgiving regimes: immigration and health care."[73] The experiences of Health Action members' attempts to access the necessary medical equipment and long-term care demonstrate the salience of immigration and health care as unforgiving. At the heart of these regimes, the ideology of public charge and its preference for able-bodied migrants characterizes Houston Health Action members as the epitome of a "bad" migrant—their wheelchairs a graphic symbol of their burdensome status. In politics and policy throughout US history, the "good" migrant, on the other hand, is an individual who only contributes to the host nation and asks for nothing in return.[74] Good migrants remain quietly in the shadows and then recede back to their home country when they are no longer productive. Most importantly, a good migrant is a worker who expects less than what they get, no matter how little. Their gratitude is illustrated by their silent acceptance of the unequal social conditions that structure their lives. In this regard, Health Action members are the antithesis of the good migrant and the embodiment of public charge. Yet it is their prominent visual representation that the organization has made central to their advocacy efforts. Their lives demand a more inclusive understanding of humanity.

Disability operates as both an experiential terrain and a framework uniquely positioned for unraveling the unforgiving inequities of immigration and health care. These regimes position undocumented migrants at the fringe of medical considerations for care and the center of deliberations for public charge. Rather than attempting to change their bodily comportment to be reincorporated into the formal medical sphere, Health Action members draw on their bodily experiences to critique and inform the infrastructure of intersecting oppressions operating throughout the US health care and immigration systems.[75] Their goal is not incorporation; it is creation, a radical refashioning of the social environment so that institutions of immigration and health care are beholden to the needs of the public, which includes undocumented migrants with disabilities.

As migrants who can no longer function as formal laborers in the national and local economy, their presence and role in the US poses fundamental questions for key social institutions. For immigration authorities, this population is a significant conundrum. The Health Action members' disability and consequent long-term health care needs classify them as within one of the few explicitly identified categories for public charge and therefore eligible for deportation. For safety net hospitals and clinics in the formal First and Second Nets, whose central purpose is to care for the underserved and vulnerable, the responsibility of ongoing care for this marginalized community also requires difficult discussions on how to care—if at all—for this clearly underserved community.

In response, Health Action members have made a conscious decision to counter this unequal infrastructure. They have made themselves visible and actively challenge health care, immigration, and disability policy in public events. The presence of Health Action members at community events and the incorporation of their experiences in policy settings speak to this relationship and subsequently counters simplistic responses that narrowly frame their illness as the problem. And, in line with their intersectional experiences, Houston Health Action explicitly critiques public charge provisions of immigration law as outdated and discriminatory against those who have disabilities.

Their continued exclusion as a patient population has accentuated their isolation from the public sphere, making them ever more vulnerable. For those undocumented migrants who are low-income and in need of long-term care, this can lead to dire circumstances. Houston Health Action members have turned this intersection on its head and exposed their own vulnerability to challenge the increasingly intertwined relationship of immigration control and health care provision.

Conclusion

Lessons from the Third Net

The Third Net is an informal, threadbare, and disconnected assortment of organizations that provide basic care to millions of migrants across the country. Crucial to the broader infrastructure of the US health care system, the Third Net serves as a convenient "dumping ground" for the formal health sector and a final resort for low-income migrants. If the configuration of the health care system remains unchallenged, the Third Net's relevance and importance will only increase over time. Public health professionals, community advocates, social scientists, and those most impacted by the health care system's infrastructure consistently emphasize the same thing: the time for bold thinking is now. As we've argued and illustrated throughout this book, Third Net practitioners' day-to-day realities provide a crucial vantage point from which to understand the purposive disarray of our health care system. In this conclusion, we synthesize their insights and experiences to highlight a few limits of the health care system and take stock of the lessons we've learned from the Third Net.

Without substantive change, the Third Net will be the future of health care for citizens. Although the scope of our research is on Third Net spaces that provide immigrant health care, it is important to recognize noncitizens' experiences as a foreshadowing of citizens' experiences. Low-income, uninsured, undocumented migrants rely on the Third Net not just because every other formal sector of the health care system has systemically failed them. They go to the Third Net because other social institutions have failed them as well. The Third Net is where migrants go for both medical *and* non-medical provisions: medicine, food, shelter, steady employment, safety, community, etc. As the current health care system continues to evolve, more and more citizens find themselves seeking these same provisions, making the Third Net more important than ever before. Thus, the lessons we take from the Third Net are important for everyone, noncitizens and citizens alike.

The Third Net imparts three central lessons for us to learn from and consider as we move further into the future. First, the health care system is not broken; it is intentionally set up this way. The Third Net is not an accident or afterthought—it plays an important role in the capitalist logic of the entire US health care infrastructure. Second, the meanings of "cost" and "care" go beyond economics and medicine, respectively. Third Net practitioners take on substantial mental and emotional labor as caregivers, and they do so in ways that recognize the broader social and political meanings of care. Third, an alternative vision of our health care system has to go beyond universal health care. Prospects like Medicare for All serve as promising starting points for health care reform, but substantive change requires a broader reconsideration about who is consistently left out and why. Together, these lessons show us that manifesting migrant health justice has required—and will continue to require—creativity and persistence. Third Net practitioners do not claim to have all the answers; nor do we. However, Third Net practitioners' experiences, stories, and day-to-day activities inform important lessons and considerations about what a health care system could be.

Lesson 1: The Health Care System Is Not "Broken"

In our courses, we invite our students to think critically about the existing health care system. As part of one lesson, we write the words "broken health care system" on the board and ask our students to raise their hand if they've ever heard the phrase. Typically, many hands shoot up. Students reflect that they've heard the phrase from politicians, news anchors, medical providers, family and friends, and other professors. Even Vermont Senator Bernie Sanders, a prominent proponent of Medicare for All, regularly refers to the health care system as "broken." But we ask our students to think further about this. We draw a line across the word "broken" and ask: "what happens if we regard the health care system as not broken?" Students think for a moment and then respond more or less the same way: if we take out the word "broken," then the implication is that the health care system is working exactly as designed and its "faults" are intentional. Extending this anecdote to the purview of

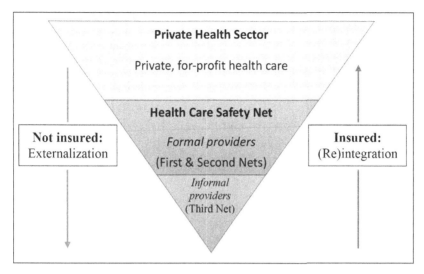

Figure c.1. US health care infrastructure: externalizing costs and reintegrating profits

this book, there is nothing accidental or unintentional about the Third Net's existence. It exists precisely because the broader health care system needs it to exist.

The US health care system is made of three interconnected parts: 1) for-profit hospitals/clinics (the private sector), 2) formal safety net providers (the First and Second Nets), and 3) informal coalitions of organizations/spaces (the Third Net) (see figure C.1). Third Net practitioners' experiences reveal a logic in this setup: it ultimately guarantees the private health care sector significant profits.

As the figure illustrates, the US health care system is characterized by a robust private sector intent on maximizing health care revenue, and every part of the health care infrastructure contributes to this in some way. As previous chapters attest, two operations occur simultaneously. First, the *formal* sector of for-profit hospitals/clinics and safety net providers ultimately relegates low-income, uninsured, undocumented migrants to the *informal* coalition of Third Net sites because, given their coverage ineligibility, they are regarded as "costly"[1] non-contributors to a health care system intent on maximizing profits. In other words, the formal sector externalizes costs associated with migrant health care to the Third Net where practitioners have varying levels of actual medical experience.[2]

At the same time, a second operation occurs wherein Third Net practitioners do everything they can to reintegrate migrants back into the formal health care safety net (i.e., the First and Second Nets), where a wider range of biomedical provisions are available. This involves creative thinking, political advocacy, and careful collaboration with formal safety net providers. The formal safety net, in turn, tries to direct patients into the private sector. Formal safety net providers are made up of public, nonprofit hospitals and clinics designed for those who cannot afford care. However, considering ongoing decreases in federal reimbursements for uncompensated care, maintaining patients' well-being within the formal health care safety net is economically challenging.[3] Thus, the fundamental purpose of the formal and informal safety net is to get patients some form of coverage (e.g., Medicaid) so that the safety net can continue to survive and patients can utilize resources in the private sector, essentially boosting the sector's profit margins with publicly financed insurance.[4] However, many undocumented migrants remain uninsurable and perpetually locked out of higher tiers of care. This is neither an accident nor an indication of a "broken" system; the disarray of care that undocumented migrants experience vis-à-vis the health care infrastructure is purposive and intentional.

The word "broken" does two important things. First, it suggests that those in positions of power made unintentional mistakes or are unaware of what they are doing. This allows lawmakers to circumvent accountability, especially in matters pertaining to migrant and racial disparities.[5] Across the political spectrum, both major political parties regularly promote immigration policies designed not to actually address undocumented migration but, rather, to bolster an already inflated Department of Homeland Security budget.[6]

When it comes to health care coverage, undocumented migrants consistently remain excluded. A frequently cited reason for this is cost.[7] Despite having lower per capita health care costs than US citizens and legal residents,[8] undocumented migrants are regularly characterized as expensive and/or a "burden" to the welfare state, and this is fundamentally about poverty governance. The language of burdensomeness breathes life into public charge laws and ideologies designed to characterize migrants as unproductive and undeserving, which, in turn, renders them as disposable and deportable. The discourse of migrant health as "costly" is so pervasive and influential that even the mere idea of expanding coverage for migrants is met with fierce resistance. To reiterate an important point, undocumented migrants' exclusion from coverage under the Affordable Care Act (ACA) in 2010 was not an oversight; it was one of the key reasons the ACA passed into law. Over a decade later, it still remains difficult to pass federal legislation designed to enable greater access to health care for immigrants. Examples include the 2021 Health Equity and Access Under the Law (HEAL) for Immigrant Families Act and the 2021 Lifting Immigrant Families Through Benefits Access Restoration (LIFT the BAR) Act. The HEAL for Immigrant Families Act would 1) extend Medicaid, Children's Health Insurance Program (CHIP), and ACA health insurance exchange access to DACA[9] recipients, 2) remove the five-year waiting period on Medicaid and CHIP for lawfully present immigrants, and 3) grant undocumented immigrants eligibility for the ACA's health insurance exchange.[10] The LIFT the BAR Act would similarly eliminate key provisions in the 1996 federal Personal Responsibility and Work Opportunity Reconciliation Act that restrict lawfully present immigrants access to a range of federal public benefit programs (e.g., Medicaid, CHIP, Supplemental Nutrition Assistance, Temporary Assistance for Needy Families).[11] Despite their merits, both Acts face a difficult path toward passage.[12] However, some states continue to make efforts to expand coverage for noncitizens, particularly pregnant women and children, but the work remains an uphill battle throughout most of the country.[13]

Second, referring to the health care system as "broken" implies that the system could meet the needs of people with a few tweaks or moderate reform. There is little evidence to support this assumption, and the COVID-19 pandemic provides an important example. As of April 2022, 12 US states still refuse to expand Medicaid,[14] a refusal that needlessly left millions of people without any coverage in the early years of the COVID-19 pandemic. The health care safety net continues to be overwhelmed by surging demands for care,[15] and reports abound of overwhelmed emergency rooms and hallways filled with patients.[16] Unequal treatment for communities of color remains an entrenched characteristic of the health care system,[17] and public health continues to be underfunded, making it difficult to disseminate time-sensitive information and resources.[18] While aspects of the COVID-19 pandemic have fluctuated across time, the United States has consistently fared the worst in terms of death and case count. At the time of this writing,[19] the United States has incurred over a million deaths, accounting for about 16% of COVID-19 deaths globally. It also has the highest number of cases in the world (over 85 million). Even if we combined the total cases of the next two high-ranking countries—India and Brazil—their case count would still be lower than the United States' case count. It's difficult to know how many more cases and deaths to expect in the United States, but trends across the first two years of the pandemic continue and we can expect these numbers to drastically increase. There's little reason to believe the United States will not hold its position as the country with the highest COVID cases and deaths worldwide. The health care system is severely strained and in need of substantial overhaul.

From the vantage point of the Third Net, the classist and racist outcomes of COVID-19 have been unsurprising because they are characteristic of a US health care infrastructure that remains centered on one thing: profit. For noncitizens and citizens alike, the health care system continues to be agonizingly expensive, and those without coverage are essentially locked out of the system. In the earlier years of the pandemic, millions lost their jobs, coinciding with the loss of employment-based insurance[20] and elevated levels of mental and emotional strain.[21] Like many Third Net organizations that regularly call for monetary donations, many uninsured and underinsured people turned to crowd-funding campaigns like GoFundMe. In the first seven months of 2020, more than 175,000 US residents created crowdfunding campaigns to offset medical costs associated with COVID-19, though 40% of these campaigns raised no money at all.[22] Medical debt is becoming an increasingly common circumstance, affecting one in 10 adults nationwide according to a 2022 Kaiser Family Foundation report.[23] The paradox is that this worst-of-times scenario coincides with a best-of-times surge in profits for various non-medical and medical sectors of society. For example, online technology corporations (e.g., Zoom, Amazon) and pharmaceutical companies (e.g., GlaxoSmithKline, Moderna, BioNTech, and Pfizer) have seen hefty stock increases and profits in the multi-billions since the start of the COVID-19 pandemic.[24] On a global level, Big Pharma continues to set high prices for a range of drugs and life-saving vaccines, exacerbating global health apartheid.[25] Hospital systems continue to merge at alarming rates, fortifying medical monopolies, driving up prices for patients, and leading to hospital closures in underserved regions (especially in the rural South).[26] Though antitrust laws exist to prevent these merging systems from becoming too large for market competition, integrations continue unabated as legal offices responsible for enforcing these laws are not able to maneuver complaints through the necessary bureaucratic channels before they expire.[27]

Third Net practitioners show us that today's health care system cannot simply be "fixed"; it must be completely transformed. Some Third Net sites like CommUnity view the health care system as fundamentally "irreparable" and in need of substantial rehaul. In the US context, "fixing" today's "broken" health care system has consistently meant expanding coverage with little to no reconfiguration of the system's existing infrastructure. Consequently, the for-profit orientation of today's health care system has remained firmly intact, leaving the Third Net with little to no formal funding. However, the problem is not necessarily that the Third Net does not receive federal funding—as stated in previous chapters, such funding would make Third Net providers beholden to state obligations. Instead, the problem is that the Third Net continues to be treated as a convenient dumping ground for patients and health care costs. Although the coalition of organizations that make up the Third Net vary in mission, philosophy, and operation, the common denominator they share is that they exist because they have to. Though Third Net organizations commonly operate in isolation from one another, they collectively make up a crucial part of the US health care infrastructure. Practitioners open their doors every day because other institutions designed to protect and nurture well-being fail (or are unable) to do so. In short, the Third Net is a necessary last resort but not a replacement for formal institutions of health care. The cases explored in our research attest to the Third Net's (sometimes life-threatening) limitations, including but not limited to unpredictable funding and labor pools, inadequate medical provisions, and charity frameworks that perpetuate racialized ideas around migrant deservingness.

Though intent on bettering the lives of those most marginalized from formal institutions of care, many Third Net practitioners explicitly note that they do not intend to do this work forever. Many of them do not call for federal funding; instead, they call for changes to the US health care and social infrastructure that make the Third Net necessary in the first place. Accomplishing these changes begins with acknowledging the Third Net's importance and explicitly recognizing its existence. Despite its significance and centrality in the entire health care infrastructure, the Third Net remains understood as "extraneous."

Lesson 2: We Need to Rethink "Costs" and "Care"

Central to the US health care infrastructure, the Third Net is where low-income migrants are "dumped" and caregiving costs are externalized. In performing the arduous and enduring work of immigrant health care, Third Net practitioners teach us that "cost" is not simply about money, and "care" is not just about medicine. When the formal sector of the health care system externalizes costs to the Third Net, it externalizes both economic and non-economic costs. The economic costs of health care and caregiving are challenging yet intuitive. Year after year, Third Net spaces have to raise millions of dollars to cover the costs of medicine, housing, food, legal fees, and expensive medical operations. The entire Third Net is funded primarily by a combination of fundraisers, charity drives, and donations. At the same time, Third Net practitioners' experiences remind us that the costs of health care and caregiving are also non-economic and include various forms of emotional, mental, and physical labor as well. The definition of "health care practitioner" expands in the Third Net. In addition to (volunteer) medical providers and support staff, practitioners within the Third Net also include community organization directors, volunteers with varying levels of medical training, members of the community, patients' family members, and even migrants themselves. With the expansion of the practitioner role comes an added layer of intimacy and connection between patients and those who provide care. Within the formal system, medical providers must adhere to medical bureaucracy and may only see patients for a few minutes at a time. Although Third Net practitioners must contend with various forms of organizational bureaucracy, their time with those in need of care is generally elongated and sometimes perpetual. This easily translates into years of emotional support (many times, until migrants die) and physical exertion (e.g., moving medical equipment; direct home care support).

Exemplifying the neoliberalization of health care, it is increasingly the case that private residents with little to no medical training are becoming responsible for life-saving tasks: procuring expensive medicines, catheters, and heavy medical beds; serving as mental health confidants without extensive training; setting up and funding informal, medically unaccredited care homes; endless fundraising; and so on. Moreover, these tasks carry the weight of empathy: caring for entire families; constantly worrying about others' physical and/or emotional well-being; and understanding that all the challenges migrant families endure are both intentional and avoidable. Third Net practitioners understand that "care" means not simply medical provision, but a collective responsibility[28] for each other.

As medical anthropologists have long acknowledged,[29] Third Net practitioners recognize illness as not simply a pathological but also a social and political construct. Given their prolonged time with patients (and sometimes entire families), Third Net practitioners experience migrant illness in deep ways. The loss of a patient in the Third Net is many times the detrimental loss of a brother, sister, parent, or child in one's own family; it's the loss of a close friend someone has been advocating for over several months or years. In some spaces (e.g., Justicia), Third Net practitioners share in a myriad of intimate experiences (e.g., quinceañeras, victories in asylum cases, the death of a family member, the birth of a newborn). In other spaces (e.g., Health Action), migrants *are* the Third Net practitioners, directly experiencing the struggles of resource mobilization and political organizing. In their view, "care" explicitly involves both life-saving medical provision and life-sustaining political advocacy.

In many ways, Third Net practitioners show us that "care" is largely about creating wellness. As experiences within the Third Net illustrate, wellness is not about the absence of pain; it's about the presence of support. This means different things in different spaces. In some spaces (e.g., Tucson's Centro de Salud; Houston's Grace in Action), support means doing whatever it takes to ensure medical provision. Within sites like CommUnity, support involves collectively rethinking what medical provision looks like. At Justicia, support can involve anything from checking a migrant's blood pressure to talking them out of suicide in the middle of night. And, in migrant-run sites like Health Action, support involves the collective construction of mutual aid networks that are otherwise prohibited or inaccessible at higher (i.e., formal) levels of care. The Third Net shows us that the opposite of illness is not health; it's wellness. Third Net practitioners recognize health as just *one* among many factors that contribute to social and political well-being.

In addition, the Third Net is made up of community-based organizations, private homes, and groups of people who understand the social and political dimensions of migrant health disparities. Some spaces (e.g., CommUnity, Centro de Salud) focus almost entirely on medical needs; others (Justicia, Houston Health Action) center on a range of social needs like housing, education, and employment. However, every Third Net site participates in some form of (in)direct political advocacy and challenges the politics of migrant exclusion. Every time the Third Net cares for a migrant, it rebukes the failure of social institutions (e.g., health care, government, education) to do their job. Interactions between immigration policy and other social policies leave undocumented migrants in a constant state of deportation and vulnerability.[30] Across the United States and other parts of the world, housing policies subject migrants to rampant homelessness.[31] Labor policies routinely fail to protect migrants from exploitation and abuse.[32] And finally, an array of federal, state, and local health care policies leave many migrants without any medical provision.[33] Through their caregiving, Third Net practitioners address and critique *all* of these areas. Thus, the Third Net's position at the bottom of the US health care infrastructure is both peculiar and significant, considering that it operates with the least formal streams of funding (e.g., insurance, government taxes) but is charged with caring for a growing volume of multiply marginalized populations (including citizens) in ways that go well beyond biomedical intervention.

Lesson 3: We Have to Go Beyond Universal Health Care

Third Net practitioners urge us to question the current infrastructure of the US health care system, and universal health care serves as a promising start. Three out of five US adults believe the government should provide some form of health coverage for all.[34] Health care spending per capita in the US is higher than in every other high-income country in the world, but the US system consistently ranks among the lowest in terms

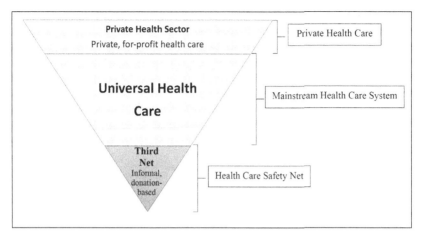

Figure C.2. Infrastructure of US health care system under a universal health care configuration

of performance.[35] Compared to Canada and Germany,[36] the US health care system leads in technological advancements but leaves a substantial portion of its residents (more than 78 million[37]) without adequate health care coverage. Had the country adopted a universal health care system prior to the COVID-19 pandemic, an estimated 338,000 lives could have been saved through the middle of 2022.[38] To date, the United States is the only high-income country without a nationwide system of care.

What impact would a universal health care system have on the Third Net? The short answer is that it depends. Third Net practitioners' experiences give us reason to suspect that under a universal health care program, the private for-profit sector would diminish, the formal health care safety net would expand in size and scope, becoming its own new mainstream system, and the Third Net itself would remain unchanged (see figure C.2). Private entities would have the option of adopting nonprofit status and participating in the program.[39] Former safety net providers would become part of the new federally funded mainstream health care system that could ostensibly offer a wider range of medical provisions, incentivizing patients to potentially use the for-profit sector less. Unlike its formal safety net counterparts, however, the Third Net would see no increase in funding or expansion of services; it would continue to run entirely on donation-based funding/resources and volunteer labor.

Although a universal health care system could offer significant benefits, Third Net practitioners' insights and experiences suggest that it would likely only serve as the first step toward addressing migrant health disparities and broader health care injustice. As figure C.2 illustrates, the Third Net would likely continue to exist under a universal health care system. At every site we visited, practitioners' stories revealed a certain logic and assumption about the Third Net's role in the health care infrastructure: it is *the* "dumping ground" for health care "costs" (as described above) and those deemed "costly." From the vantage point of the Third Net, this is unlikely to change under a universal health care system. Proposals for universal health care programs vary but essentially share the promise of offering coverage to "all Americans."[40] Undocumented migrants, among other multiply marginalized groups, may not be included in the category of "American." Third Net practitioners have learned to anticipate this and assume that discussions about migrant health care would remain contentious or conversation non-starters. Health analysts agree: "Eligibility for benefits [under a universal health care program] is . . . likely to be politically controversial, particularly with regard to undocumented immigrants."[41] Migrants continue to be framed as "public charges" or "burdens" to society. Even though noncitizens incur significantly fewer health care costs than their citizen counterparts,[42] politicians across the political spectrum continue to characterize them as "costly," justifying 1) the continual existence of a Third Net and 2) noncitizens' relegation (i.e., "dumping") into the Third Net. The Third Net repeatedly reminds us that "universal" does not necessarily mean "everyone." Noncitizens already have varied levels of access to the formal health care system, but as the Third Net clearly reveals, "health access" is not the same thing as "health justice." This leaves us with the question, what does health justice look like?

Like Third Net practitioners, we acknowledge that we don't know all the answers. The cases explored in this book offer a proximate understanding of the Third Net and its role within the broader health care infrastructure, but there is still plenty that we don't know. And, as variation across the Third Net illustrates, there is no single right way to do things. Every Third Net site operates with a different philosophy of care, a unique internal infrastructure of their own, a particular set of health system critiques, and distinct ideas about what a future health care system could look like. Despite their heterogeneity, however, the organizations that collectively make up the Third Net share an important consideration—a starting point, if you will—about what "health justice" could involve: their visions of health care consistently begin with low-income undocumented migrants in mind. Practitioners from CommUnity articulate this explicitly, asking us—scholars, students, policymakers, activists, health providers, and so on—to consider the question: what does a health care system look like when it *begins* with the most marginalized populations in mind? The allure of this question is that it inspires different answers across time and space. It also encourages us to think deeply about all the sociopolitical influences at work outside of *and* within the health care system's infrastructure, particularly factors that directly impact low-income undocumented migrants: racism, patriarchy, xenophobia, ableism, etc. Over recent years, proposals for universal health care *end* with considerations about migrant health care—in the popular imagination, migrants will receive whatever is "left over." From the vantage point of the Third Net, however, universal health care can only be "universal" when it *begins* with considerations about migrant health care.

The greatest paradox about the Third Net's position at the bottom of the US health care infrastructure is that it comes closer to universal coverage than its formal counterparts. In general terms, universal health care is a publicly financed system where everyone contributes to the health and well-being of others. This is exactly what the Third Net does. Every Third Net site is financed by a broader public that believes in the aim of providing care to everyone. In lieu of taxes, the Third Net receives material and monetary donations and hours of dedicated labor. People across the nation and the globe contribute to the Third Net precisely because they believe the simple yet profound notion that other people should be okay. Universal coverage sounds less "radical" when we recognize that the Third Net has been doing this for decades, dedicating its entire existence to the well-being of the most marginalized populations in the country. The Third Net is significantly limited in terms of meeting everyone's needs. Nevertheless, it provides us crucial considerations for imagining what an alternative health care system could look like.

ACKNOWLEDGMENTS

This book is a collaborative effort and required the support and generosity of so many. Foremost in our minds are the many dedicated members of organizations and health care providers in the Third Net, and beyond, who shared their valuable time and knowledge with us. We are also thankful to our manuscript workshop participants, Sofya Aptekar, Heide Castañeda, and Sameena Mulla, for their insightful comments, as well as Jennifer Reich and the two anonymous reviewers whose suggestions significantly improved our book. In addition, we were so fortunate to have the steadfast support of Ilene Kalish, executive editor at NYU Press. We could not imagine a smoother publication process.

Lisa Sun-Hee Park would like to acknowledge the support of friends and scholars whose kindness and encouragement propelled this project over the years. The initial idea for this research took root at the University of Minnesota, Twin Cities (UMN). Lisa is grateful to colleagues in the Asian American Studies program, the Department of Sociology, and beyond, for providing a generous intellectual space. In particular, Lisa is thankful for the opportunity to meet Erin Hoekstra and Anthony Jimenez as graduate students at UMN. Very early on in the research process, it was clear that their contributions exceeded that of a research assistant and their transition to co-authors was nearly automatic. This book would not exist without them and its strengths derive from its collective origins. At the University of California, Santa Barbara, Lisa found a wonderful community of scholars across multiple departments, particularly in Asian American Studies. In addition, the writing sessions with Sofya Aptekar and Miriam Ticktin, and another with Adria Imada, were incredibly valuable in meeting the deadlines for this manuscript. And no acknowledgment would be complete without thanking David Pellow and Jin Pellow for all that they do. Finally, Lisa would like to acknowledge the thoughtful comments from participants at presentations delivered at the annual conference of the American Sociological Association and the Association for Asian American Studies.

Erin expresses her gratitude for the community of academics, activists, colleagues, and family and friends who have provided their guidance and encouragement during the research and writing process. This book would not have been possible without the institutional and financial support of the Department of Sociology at the University of Minnesota, the Bilinski Foundation, and the Anna Welsch Bright Research Fellowship. Erin navigated the research and writing journey with the support, mentorship, and friendship of many colleagues at the University of Minnesota, the Center for Comparative Immigration Studies at the University of California-San Diego, and Marquette University. Working with Lisa Sun-Hee Park and Anthony Jimenez has been, by far, the highlight of her professional career. Their support and camaraderie are invaluable, and they continue to inspire her as scholars and friends. The mentorship of Teresa Gowan, her keen ethnographic eye, attention to the craft of writing, and constant encouragement to "be bold, be wrong!" have shaped Erin as a scholar. The last thing Erin expected to find in academia was a partner, much less a partner in life and comrade in struggle as supportive as Raphi Rechitsky. He has believed in her when she did not and continually reminds her that her work matters. When Erin despairs that her daughter is inheriting a less just and equitable world, Raisa Hoekstra-Rechitsky's feisty spirit, defiant joie de vivre, and unbridled curiosity are a source of abundant joy and provide hope for the future. She is more than grateful to share life with these two wonderful humans. Erin's deep admiration and gratitude go to the volunteers and patients at the CommUnity Clinic of Phoenix and other Third Net organizations and activists in Arizona, providing medical care to migrants in the borderlands and fostering radical hospitality in the face of state repression. They took her in, shared their knowledge and perspectives, and continue to work tirelessly to cultivate mutual aid and community solidarity.

Anthony Jimenez is deeply grateful for the institutional and personal support he received during the research and writing stages of this book project. His ethnographic fieldwork would not have been possible without the support of the University of Minnesota's Sociology Department and Interdisciplinary Center for the Study of Global Change, Rice University's Kinder Institute for Urban Research, and the Ford Foundation.

Anthony is especially indebted to his co-authors, Lisa Sun-Hee Park and Erin Hoekstra, for their unyielding support. With them, this journey has been filled with countless hours of laughter, learning, and personal growth. Anthony's colleagues and friends from the University of Minnesota, North Carolina State University, and the Rochester Institute of Technology have also been a constant source of support, providing mentorship, guidance, and numerous opportunities for brainstorming and peer review. In addition to his family, Anthony is also especially grateful for the love and unyielding support of his partner, Wenjie Liao. Every time self-doubt, exhaustion, or feelings of defeat knocked Anthony down, Wenjie was there to lift him back up. Lastly, Anthony is grateful for the generosity and courage of migrants and volunteers at Justicia y Paz. Experiences shared within Justicia y Paz and the wider Houston community constantly reminded Anthony that people can accomplish incredible things when they work together. Every challenge was met with amazing wit, perseverance, and patience. Every victory—no matter how large or small—was embraced with love, celebration, and solidarity. Anthony is forever thankful for the opportunity to grow with and learn from Justicia y Paz and its astonishing network of supporters.

Finally, we would like to acknowledge that portions of this book appear in earlier publications. Portions of chapter 1 appeared in Erin Hoekstra and Anthony Jimenez's "Versatile Brokerage: Immigrant-Provider Relationships in the Third Net of the U.S. Healthcare System" in the *Journal of Ethnic and Migration Studies* (2023). Portions of chapter 3 appeared in Erin Hoekstra's "'Not a Free Version of a Broken System': Medical Humanitarianism and Immigrant Health Justice in the United States" in *Social Science & Medicine*, vol. 285 (2021). And sections of chapter 4 appeared in Lisa S. Park, Anthony Jimenez, and Erin Hoekstra's "Decolonizing the U.S. Health Care System: Undocumented and Disabled After the Affordable Care Act" in *Health Tomorrow: Interdisciplinarity and Internationality*, vol. 5, no. 1 (2017).

NOTES

INTRODUCTION

1 Lewin and Altman 2000.

2 Ashley Carse (2016, 27) defines "infrastructure" as having two fundamental characteristics: first, it is "a collective term: a singular noun that, like system and network, denotes a plurality of integrated parts. Second, those collective parts are understood to support some higher-order project."

3 We use the term "migrant" to describe people and populations of foreign birth or citizenship, or those who moved from another country for temporary purposes or to settle long-term. The term "immigrant" refers to policies and practices related to the control of national borders.

4 According to the US Census, 44% of US immigrants (19.8 million people) were Hispanic/Latino in 2019, 27% were Asian, 10% were Black, 15% reported some other race, and approximately 2% reported having two or more races. See Rosenblum and Ruiz Soto 2015 (Migration Policy Institute).

5 Noncitizens include legal permanent residents ("green card" holders), refugees, asylees, and others with temporary or permanent visas, as well as undocumented migrants.

6 Migration Policy Institute (Rosenblum and Ruiz Soto 2015). Undocumented migrants are foreign born and reside in the US without authorization. This includes those who entered without authorization and those who entered with authorization and overstayed their visa.

7 Documented elderly (over age 65) migrants living in the US for over five years have access to additional health coverage through Medicare. And, with the passage of the ACA, documented elderly migrants not eligible for Medicare can purchase private health insurance in the insurance exchange/marketplace and receive income-based tax credits to offset the cost if they do not qualify for government- or employer-sponsored coverage.

8 Kaiser Commission on Key Facts 2013.

9 Kaiser Family Foundation 2022. The higher uninsured rate for documented migrants reflects limited access to private employer-sponsored coverage, eligibility restrictions for public health insurance programs, and fear and confusion about their eligibility for health care and its impact on their immigration status.

10 "Immigrants, Health Care and Lies," September 10, 2009.

11 A. L. Campbell and Shore-Sheppard 2020, 1.

12 Sances and Clinton 2019.
13 Henderson and Hillygus 2011; Tesler 2012.
14 Staiti, Hurley, and Katz 2006.
15 This figure is adapted from the work of Rice and colleagues (2013). The Commonwealth Fund is a private foundation that supports independent research on health care and provides grants to improve health care practice and policy. www.commonwealthfund.org.
16 Berchick, Barnett, and Upton 2019.
17 Of those privately insured, 81.9% are through their employer. A small portion (2.6%) of private insurance is comprised of TRICARE, a regionally managed health care program for active duty and retired members of the uniformed serves, their families, and survivors (Berchick, Barnett, and Upton 2019, 2).
18 FQHCs are community-based nonprofit health care providers that receive funds from the federal Human Resources & Services Administration to provide primary care services in underserved areas. Their fees are sliding scale based on one's ability to pay.
19 See Tikkanen, Roosa, et al. 2020. www.commonwealthfund.org.
20 See Sutton et al. 2016.
21 Please note that given the focus of this study, figure I.4 represents the safety net health care tiers disproportionately large in comparison to the private health care sector. This is to illustrate greater detail within the safety net, and its location below the private sector.
22 See Lewin and Altman 2000.
23 There are two main Medicaid compensation systems: the Disproportionate Share Hospital (DSH) payment program for hospitals and the FQHC program for federally funded health centers.
24 See Starfield et al. 1994. See also hospital quality indicators provided by Centers for Medicare & Medicaid Services: www.medicare.gov.
25 "Death Caused by Removal," New York Times, August 10, 1891; cited in Abel 2011, 791.
26 Ansell and Schiff (1987) contend that laws against patient dumping are inadequate in defining such terms as "emergency" and "patient stability" and that monitoring and enforcement of existing laws and the guidelines of the American College of Emergency Physicians are severely lacking.
27 "Medically indigent" refers to patients who are uninsured or underinsured and cannot cover the cost of their care. See Nutter 1987.
28 See MacKenzie et al. 2012, 1790.
29 Nessel 2012; Park 2018.
30 Enfield and Sklar 1988, 561.
31 See Himmelstein et al. 1984.
32 Schiff et al. 2019.
33 See Kellermann and Hackman 1988.
34 Enfield and Sklar 1988, 585. This action also disadvantages patients by inferring consent for the transfer, which then absolves the transferring hospital for

violating any anti-dumping statute and the patient has no cause of action against the hospital.

35 Ibid.
36 Kellermann and Hackman 1988, 1291.
37 Ibid. This figure excludes St. Jude Children's Research Hospital.
38 Ibid.
39 Koetting 1989.
40 Enfield and Sklar 1988, 562.
41 Ibid., 592.
42 Star 1999, 377.
43 Appel, Anand, and Gupta 2018, 4.
44 Anand 2017, vii.
45 Ibid., 11.
46 Ibid., 13.
47 See Piven and Cloward 1971; Soss, Fording, and Schram 2011; Wacquant 2009; Seim 2017.
48 See Weber 1948.
49 See Lipsky 1980.
50 See US Citizenship and Immigration Services (USCIS), www.uscis.gov.
51 See Patricia Hill Collins's critique of this image in *Black Feminist Thought*, 2008.
52 Pre-enactment migrants are those who entered the United States before August 22, 1996, when the welfare reform bill was signed into law, and post-enactment migrants are those who entered on or after August 22, 1996. Both of these categories of migrants are documented and "legally" reside in the US.
53 See Morse et al. 1998.
54 De Genova 2004; Jimenez 2022.
55 Bacong and Menjívar 2021, 1097.
56 See Menjívar et al. 2018; Gee et al. 2019.
57 Citing Karthick Ramakrishnan, co-director of AAPI Data, in V. Williams 2017.
58 Bacong and Menjívar 2021, 1098.
59 Ornelas, Yamanis, and Ruiz 2020, 289.
60 Vernice et al. 2020, 15.
61 Ibid., 16.
62 Castañeda et al. 2015, 377.
63 Krieger 1994; 2001.
64 D. R. Williams 1999.
65 Takeuchi 2016; Takeuchi and Gage 2003.
66 Phelan, Link, and Tehranifar 2010; Phelan and Link 2015.
67 Kawachi and Kennedy 1997; 1999.
68 Viruell-Fuentes, Miranda, and Abdulrahim 2012; 2103.
69 A. L. Campbell and Shore-Sheppard 2020, 1.
70 See A. L. Campbell and Shore-Sheppard 2020 and Levy, Ying, and Bagley 2020 for an overview of ACA implementation.

71 Howland et al. 2014.
72 Kaiser Commission on Key Facts 2013.
73 Goldman, Smith, and Sood 2006.
74 H. S. Brown, Wilson, and Angel 2015, 997.
75 See Felland et al. 2016.
76 Ibid., 7.
77 Ibid., 59.
78 These reductions were initially set to occur from 2014 through 2020 but were amended by a series of laws and delayed to begin in 2024 through 2027. See Congressional Research Service 2021.
79 Marrow and Joseph 2015.
80 Van Natta et al. 2019, 49–55.
81 Ibid., 50.
82 Associated Press 2012.
83 Cheney and Millman 2013; Norman 2013.
84 Families USA 2017.
85 Baxter 2014.
86 Ibid.
87 Alltucker 2015.
88 Ibid.
89 Barnett and Berchick 2017.
90 White 2017.
91 Kaiser Family Foundation 2022.
92 Norris 2022.
93 Ibid.
94 Ramirez et al. 2021; Cox et al. 2016.
95 United States Census Bureau 2021; Stacker 2022.
96 State of Arizona Office of the Auditor General, 2009; see also Kwok 2020.
97 Harris County Healthcare Alliance 2016.
98 For more information, please see the Texas Medical Center website, www .texasmedicalcenter.org.
99 Harris Health System 2018.
100 Ibid.
101 Finegold et al. 2021; Ye and Rodriguez 2021. There is some variation in reports of the number of uninsured nonelderly adults in 2016, after implementation of the ACA. For instance, A. L. Campbell and Shore-Sheppard (2020, 1) note that determining exact numbers is challenging but that simple estimates derived from extending pre-existing trends in uninsured rates show that more than 18 million gained insurance in 2016 due to the ACA. Finegold's estimate is closer to 20 million.
102 Ye and Rodriguez 2021.
103 Harvey 2020, 1.
104 Lakoff 2020, 1.

105 Adhikari et al. 2020.
106 See Yudell et al. 2020.
107 See www.cdc.gov.
108 After an initial visit, we pulled Albuquerque as a research site given its unique history and politics of race and immigration. Concerns regarding immigration and migrant health were expressed in significantly distinct ways from neighboring states and it became evident that New Mexico should be studied separately, with careful attention to its past and present colonial context and American Indian heritage.
109 All of the ethnographic sites are given pseudonyms.
110 See Molloy, Walker, and Lakeman 2017.
111 Braun and Clarke 2006.

1. PHILOSOPHIES OF CARE
1 Burt 2000; 2004; 2005; Fernandez and Gould 1994; Gould and Fernandez 1989; Marsden 1982; Small 2009; Stovel, Golub, and Milgrom 2011; Stovel and Shaw 2012.
2 Community health workers (CHWs) and navigators under the Affordable Care Act have highlighted the importance of street-level bureaucrats in facilitating migrant access to health care and emphasized the institutionalization of brokerage relationships under the current health system. CHWs and navigators have played a central role in helping those previously uninsured navigate the bureaucratic channels to enroll in coverage through the new health marketplaces. In doing so, CHWs and navigators act as "brokers," connecting their low-income, marginalized community members to health care coverage and access (López-Sanders 2017a; 2017b). As liaisons primarily between uninsured migrant patients and the medical system, these health care brokers serve as both patient representatives and gatekeepers to medical resources, providing linguistic support, identifying insurance alternatives, and culling information from migrant networks (López-Sanders 2017a; Okie 2007; Shi et al. 2009; Viladrich 2005). In this way, they link newly insurable patients with the health care safety net, or the second tier of the health system in the US. For more discussion of brokerage and street-level bureaucrats, see Aptekar 2020; Belabas and Gerrits 2017; Borrelli 2019; Edlins and Larrison 2020; M. Kelly 1994; Lamphere 2005; Lipsky 1980; 2010; Maynard-Moody and Musheno 2000; Portes and Sensenbrenner 1993.
3 These semi-formal relationships between Third Net organizations and volunteers and the mainstream health system vary depending on state and local policy contexts around health and immigration. For instance, Harris County's Gold Card program has facilitated access to health care in the mainstream system for uninsured people regardless of immigration status, and Third Net organizations like Justicia y Paz, discussed later in this chapter, are able to provide letters for migrants' applications to satisfy the residence requirement.

4 Hoekstra and Jimenez 2023.
5 D. E. Smith 1976; Darnell 2010; Taylor 1979; Nibbe 2012.
6 Alondra Nelson 2011; Bassett 2016; 2019; Frierson 2020; P. Brown et al. 2004.
7 D. E. Smith and Seymour 1997, 156.
8 Nibbe 2012.
9 DeVoe 2008.
10 Taylor 1979.
11 Ibid.; Kemble 2000.
12 San Augustine's is a pseudonym for the FQHC.
13 Picarda 2014; Bryson, McGuiness, and Ford 2002.
14 Monetary and in-kind donations to nonprofit organizations are tax-deductible and therefore introduce a financial motivation in addition to altruistic and moral motivations.
15 Pullan 2019.
16 H. W. Munson 1930.
17 Starr 1982; S. D. Watson 2009.
18 Starr 1982.
19 Ibid.
20 D'Agostini 2019; V. J. Munson 2017.
21 Becerra 2016; McDowell and Wonders 2009; A. Maldonado 2013; Romero 2011.
22 Braveman et al. 2011; Christopher and Caruso 2015; McKay and Taket 2020; Marmot 2021.
23 Kline 2019; Rhodes et al. 2015.
24 Hoekstra 2021.
25 This framing of their work and CCP's health care provision will be further addressed in chapter 3.
26 Hoekstra 2021.
27 Day 1952; Deines 2008; McKanan 2008; Morton and Saltmarsh 1997.
28 Harris Health System 2000.
29 Jimenez 2021.
30 Hoekstra and Jimenez 2023.
31 Tolentino 2020; see also Arnold 2020.
32 Spade 2020a, 136.
33 National Humanities Center 2009.
34 New Hampshire Bureau of Labor 1894; see also Aderath 2020.
35 Aderath 2020.
36 Spade 2020a; 2020b.
37 Gammage 2021; Spade 2020b.
38 The exact citation has been omitted to protect the organization's and volunteer's identities.
39 Ibid.
40 Ibid.

41 Some organizations that do not become 501c3 organizations themselves are still able to access funding through a fiscal sponsorship. This is when another designated 501c3 organization acts as their sponsor and provides some additional oversight and resources to the organization.

2. ALL ROADS LEAD TO THE THIRD NET

1 Coy 2001; Deines 2008; McKanan 2008.
2 The Harris Health System was formerly known as the Harris County Hospital District. Harris Health System 2018.
3 Monday and Porsa 2020.
4 Beyer 2015.
5 Lewin and Altman 2000.
6 Rosenblum and Ruiz Soto 2015.
7 Houses of hospitality are community-run organizations that provide care to a range of populations including migrants, sex workers, and the homeless (Stock 2014, 151).
8 Catholic Worker Movement 2023.
9 It is unclear to what degree Justicia y Paz is under threat. The notion that urban developers see the organization as a missed opportunity for development is based on volunteer speculation.
10 For example, see Brill 2015; Geyman 2021; Okie 2007.
11 See Waitzkin and Jasso-Aguilar 2015.
12 The Federal 1986 Emergency Medical Treatment and Active Labor act prohibits patient dumping.
13 Cervantes and Menjívar 2020; Jimenez 2021; Van Natta et al. 2019.
14 Bonilla-Silva 2020.
15 Schaffer 2021, 46.
16 Aptekar 2020; Lipsky 2010.
17 Coughlin et al. 2012; Islam et al. 2015; Phillips and Fitzsimons 2015.
18 Gordon 2005; Sears 1999.
19 Chomsky 1999; Waitzkin and Jasso-Aguilar 2015; Waitzkin 2000; 2005.
20 Seim 2017; Soss, Fording, and Schram 2011.
21 See Park 2018.
22 Bourdieu 1991.
23 Boehrer 2003.
24 McKanan 2008; Morton and Saltmarsh 1997.
25 Stock 2014, 151.
26 Coy 2001; Deines 2008; Zwick and Zwick 2005.
27 Morton and Saltmarsh 1997.
28 Day 1952, 150.
29 Jimenez 2021.
30 Boehrer 2003; Morton and Saltmarsh 1997.
31 Catholic Worker Movement 2023.

32 Larry, Margaret's late husband, used to give these talks. After he became ill, however, Margaret started delivering them: "My husband gave the talks for years and years. He used to be a priest years ago and . . . knows how to give talks that reach people's hearts in churches. So, he doesn't give the talks anymore but we use his format [laughs]." This quote is from an interview before Larry passed away.

33 For example, see Jimenez and Collins 2017.

34 H. Murray 1990, 79.

35 Segers 1978, 228.

36 Maniscalco 2020.

37 Asad 2020; Cervantes and Menjívar 2020; Joseph 2017; Okie 2007; Park 2011; Portes, Fernández-Kelly, and Light 2012; Van Natta et al. 2019; Viladrich 2012; T. Watson 2014.

38 Zwick and Zwick 2005.

39 Foucault 1975; Holmes 2012.

40 Cervantes and Menjívar 2020; Jimenez 2021; Van Natta 2019.

41 Matt. 14:13–21.

42 Andrulis and Siddiqui 2011.

43 See Jahnke et al. 2015, 1; Kelley and Tipirneni 2018. Josh, an official from Harris Health, explains: "the 1115 waiver is a federal program that allows us to receive money for uncompensated care and then also for innovative programs to improve access." The waiver comes with two different pools of funding: 1) uncompensated care (UC) and 2) Delivery System Reform Incentive Payments (DSRIP). The UC pool, it was presumed, would make up for diminishing federal reimbursements: "I think there's a sense about the hospital system that they'll just use the 1115 waiver projects to offset their own uncompensated care." The DSRIP pool, on the other hand, would incentivize innovation and health district growth. Charles, another official with Harris Health, summarizes: "DSRIPs are like innovative projects to produce greater efficiency." DSRIP programs "pay incentive payments to hospitals and other safety-net providers for reaching preestablished milestones that improve quality and cost of care."

44 People in the coverage gap make too much money (above 43% of the federal poverty level; $8,935 for a family of three) to qualify for Medicaid but not enough (below 100% of the federal poverty level; $12,140 for individuals) to qualify for Marketplace premium tax credits.

45 This figure combines those below the current Medicaid eligibility, those in the coverage gap, and those who are currently eligible for Marketplace coverage (i.e., with income levels between 100% and 138% of the federal poverty level) (Garfield, Orgera, and Damico 2021).

46 Rosenblum and Ruiz Soto 2015.

47 The relationship between Justicia y Paz and Harris Health is generative. A coalition of eight organizations affiliated with Harris Health operates solely with the purpose of enrolling new Medicaid beneficiaries. However, ineligible individuals (i.e., undocumented migrants) are not part of their focus. This became a pattern. We

met with community health worker trainers, eligibility and media relations specialists, and safety net administrators, and every time we asked about health care for undocumented immigrants, the conversations slowed. When we followed up with questions about long-term care for undocumented migrants, the conversations stopped.

48 Andrulis and Siddiqui 2011.

49 Park 2018.

50 Gastroenterologists generally treat individuals with digestive problems.

51 Cervantes and Menjívar 2020; Van Natta 2019; Jimenez 2021.

52 Justicia y Paz's newsletter—the *Houston Catholic Worker*—serves as the organization's primary form of information dissemination and request for funding. Volunteers and the organization's founders—Margaret and her late husband Larry—generally share stories in the newsletter about what it's like to be a Catholic Worker. Migrants who contribute to the newsletter generally recount their experiences on route to and within the United States.

53 Morton and Saltmarsh 1997.

54 Genworth 2020.

55 See Jimenez 2021.

56 Ibid.

57 Jimenez 2021; Park 2011.

58 The US health care system adopts a business model that centers on maximizing profits, or what scholars call a "medical industrial complex" (Grouse 2014; Relman 1980).

59 For some time, individuals received an actual Gold Card verifying their approval for the program. Now, the Harris Health System simply provides patients with a paper indicating that they were approved for the Gold Card program.

60 Harris Health System 2000.

61 Ibid.

62 The Gold Card is not health insurance or recognized as an official form of health coverage. The program is intended to supplement health insurance. Between 2010 and 2018, individuals who had a Gold Card but no form of officially recognized health insurance still incurred a tax penalty under the Affordable Care Act's individual mandate. Since 2019, this tax penalty—also referred to as a "shared responsibility payment"—no longer applies (HealthCare.Gov 2022).

63 The program separates levels of assistance into five tiers or "levels of financial responsibility." See Harris Health System 2000.

64 Heyman, Núñez, and Talavera 2009; Portes, Light, and Fernández-Kelly 2009; Portes, Fernández-Kelly, and Light 2012.

65 Harris Health System 2020.

66 Ibid.

67 See Jimenez 2021.

68 Beitler et al. 2020; Ranney, Griffeth, and Jha 2020.

69 Ritzer 2021.

70 The number of partner organizations may have changed since the time of our study.

71 Jimenez 2021.
72 Cervantes and Menjívar 2020; Jimenez 2021; Van Natta 2019; 2023.
73 Varsanyi et al. 2012.
74 For example, see Marrow and Joseph 2015.
75 Harris Health System 2020.
76 Klineberg et al. 2014.
77 Justicia y Paz operates as part of the New Sanctuary Movement.
78 A range of experiences are detailed in the newsletters, including but not limited to hardships while crossing the border, sexual violence, family separation, domestic abuse, and medical challenges.
79 Half of this food goes to another Justicia y Paz–affiliated space for a separate Thursday morning food distribution.
80 Like other Food Bank goods, half of the turkeys go to Justicia y Paz's main house, and the other half go to another Justicia y Paz–affiliated space.
81 This contrasts sharply with spaces inspired by traditional Catholicism, wherein priests serve as the direct intermediaries of God and prescribe parishioners' actions (Segers 1978).
82 Translated from Spanish.
83 Jimenez 2022.
84 Muers (2021, 44) explains that the line—"you always have the poor with you"— "gives divine sanction, not merely to the continued existence of economic and class division, but also to the theological and moral judgment of 'the poor' by a privileged group . . . who can prescribe the correct response to poverty."
85 Stock 2014, 151.
86 Navarro 2020.
87 Fields and Hodkinson 2018; Nethercote 2020; Wetzstein 2017.
88 Niles et al. 2020; M. D. Smith and Wesselbaum 2020.

3. BEYOND CHARITY

1 CommUnity Clinic of Phoenix is a pseudonym. All names of individuals—both volunteers and patients—are also pseudonyms.
2 This semi-secrecy is a common trait among many Third Net organizations. Given the nature of their work, these organizations may choose, like CommUnity, to maintain a certain level of covertness in their operations. However, this secrecy in terms of not publicizing their work with a sign on the outside of the building exists alongside a robust online presence through social media and organizational websites as well as a strong referral and word-of-mouth networking among the communities that the organization serves.
3 Berk and Schur 2001; Hacker et al. 2012; C. Z. Maldonado et al. 2013; Page-Reeves et al. 2013.
4 Kline 2017; 2019; Portes, Fernández-Kelly, and Light 2012.
5 List 2011; Pellegrino 1999; Smith-Carrier 2020.
6 Kemble 2000, 419.

7   Hoekstra 2021.

8   Ibid.

9   We refer to immigrant health justice in this chapter when discussing policies of immigrant health care and when relating the language used by CommUnity Clinic of Phoenix. We refer to migrant health justice when discussing the broader concept of health justice for migrant patients.

10 A pseudonym.

11 Aguirre 2012; K. M. Campbell 2011; Magaña and Lee 2013; Nill 2011.

12 SB 1070 (or the Support Our Law Enforcement and Safe Neighborhoods Act), passed by the Arizona legislature in 2010, is the controversial policy that became known as the "show me your papers" law. SB 1070 originally had four main provisions, three of which were eventually struck down in legal battles as unconstitutional. The fourth provision that remained requires law enforcement to determine the immigration status of anyone that they stop, detain, or arrest if there is "reasonable suspicion" that they may be undocumented. The law was subject to many legal challenges and has been critiqued for essentially legalizing racial profiling.

13 To protect the anonymity of the clinic, the documentary film is not specifically cited.

14 Hoekstra 2021.

15 Garcés, Scarinci, and Harrison 2006; Hacker et al. 2012.

16 Third Net organizations that access government and foundation grant funding face the challenges and pressures of delivering outcomes to external entities. In order to stress the volume of their work (under what CCP would describe as the "quantity" model of care), these organizations may make the strategic decision to highlight the number of monthly and annual patient visits to stress the volume of the demand for the care that they provide. CCP critiqued this approach to accounting as impersonal and another indicator of differences to their immigrant health justice approach to emphasizing "quality" care.

17 The exact citation has been omitted to protect the organization's identity.

18 For a discussion of structural vulnerability, see Quesada, Hart, and Bourgois 2011; Holmes 2011.

19 An A1C of 6.5 or higher means that someone has diabetes, while an A1C higher than 8 indicates diabetes that is not well-controlled. For a CCP patient or poten-tial patient, an A1C this high would be a reason for alarm, as the patient would not have access to health care and diabetes medication and would be at risk for a host of more serious secondary health issues as a result.

20 For a discussion of structural violence, see Farmer 2004.

21 Adebowale and Rao 2020; Islam and Ahmed 2021; Page-Reeves et al. 2013; Viruell-Fuentes, Miranda, and Abdulrahim 2012.

22 Evashwick 1989, 30.

23 For more information about naturopathic medicine, see Bradley et al. 2019; Elder 2013.

4. CHALLENGING PUBLIC CHARGE

1 This is a pseudonym.

2 Houston Health Action's infrastructure differs from other mutual aid organizations in its executive director position. The membership voted for this leadership position so that a particular member, who had prior experience as a labor organizer and one of the few members bilingual in Spanish and English, could serve as the spokesperson, especially in the early stages of its founding.

3 Report from organization's website posted on January 28, 2019, 6.

4 See Espiritu and Duong 2022; Minich 2016; Schalk 2017.

5 Interview with author, May 2014.

6 USCIS 2009.

7 Park 2005; 2011; Hutchinson 1987; Evans 1987; Fairchild 2005.

8 Gardner 2009, 89.

9 Fairchild 2005; Hutchinson 1987; Higham 1976.

10 Park 2005; 2011; Okie 2007; Viladrich 2012.

11 Baynton 2005, 41.

12 Fairchild 2005, 14.

13 Evans 1987.

14 USCIS 2009. "Long-term care" refers to a broad set of paid and unpaid services for people who need assistance with daily living activities due to a chronic illness or physical or mental disability. It can also include medical and therapeutic treatment (see Feder, Komisar, and Niefeld 2000).

15 Public charge determinations also occur during medical screening for legal permanent resident status. See Aptekar 2020.

16 Park 2011.

17 See California State Auditor 1999.

18 Exec. Order No. 12,356, 8 CFR 103, 212, 213, 214, [237], and 248 [CIS No. 2499–10; DHS Docket No. USCIS-2010–0012] (2017).

19 Hauslohner and Ross 2017.

20 Exec. Order No. 12,356, 8 CFR 103, 212, 213, 214, [237], and 248 [CIS No. 2499–10; DHS Docket No. USCIS-2010–0012] (2017).

21 Ku and Bruen 2013.

22 Immigrant Legal Resource Center 2022, 1.

23 Bernstein et al. 2020.

24 Interview with author, May 2014.

25 Interview with author, May 2014.

26 This one paid employee is the executive director.

27 Interview with author, May 2014.

28 Report from organization's website posted on January 28, 2019, 5.

29 Ibid.

30 Ibid.

31 Stone 2001, 97.

32 Ibid.
33 Interview with author, May 2014.
34 Kennedy, Greene, and Saint 2013.
35 Interview with author, May 2014.
36 Interview with author, May 2014.
37 Workers Defense Project 2013.
38 Passel and Cohn 2016.
39 Kovic 2014, 18.
40 Seabury, Terp, and Boden 2017.
41 Ackerman 2011.
42 Rice 2011.
43 Ibid.
44 Ackerman 2011.
45 Kaye, Harrington, and LaPlante 2010, 19.
46 Ibid.
47 Levine et al. 2010, 117.
48 Feder, Komisar, and Niefeld 2000, 41.
49 Those "in the community" are distinguished from those in nursing homes. Komisar and Niefeld 2000, cited in Feder, Komisar, and Niefeld 2000, 41.
50 Feder, Komisar, and Niefeld 2000, 50.
51 Interview with author, May 2015.
52 Interview with author, May 2014.
53 Report from organization's website posted in 2013.
54 Cited from media report on organization published in 2020.
55 See Spade 2020a.
56 Ibid., 2.
57 Chen 2020.
58 Interview with author, May 2014.
59 Interview with author, May 2015.
60 Cited in Ticktin 2021.
61 Ibid.
62 Clare 1999.
63 Shakespeare 2013.
64 Ibid., 215.
65 Ibid.
66 Ibid., 218.
67 See Crow 1996.
68 Wendell 2013.
69 Wiener 2013, 834.
70 Ibid., 831.
71 See Kaye, LaPlante, and Harrington 2009.
72 See Levy, Ying, and Bagley 2020, 54.
73 Nessel 2012, 63.

74 Park 2011.
75 Collins 2008.

CONCLUSION
1 This point is elaborated in a later section.
2 Jimenez 2021.
3 Jimenez 2021; Wallace et al. 2013.
4 Sociologist Howard Waitzkin (2000) calls this the "private-public contradiction."
5 Ebert, Liao, and Estrada 2020; Estrada, Ebert, and Liao 2020; Forman 2004; Forman and Lewis 2006; Mueller 2017; Mueller and Issa 2016.
6 For more info about the immigration-industrial complex, see Golash-Boza 2009. In a recent example, the Biden Administration's 2022 fiscal year budget allocates the Department of Homeland Security over $52 billion in discretionary funding. See "FY 2022 Budget-in-Brief," www.dhs.gov.
7 Park 2011.
8 Park, Jimenez, and Hoekstra 2017.
9 Deferred Action for Childhood Arrivals (DACA) is a US immigration policy that allows individuals who came to the United States as children to apply for temporary renewable protection from deportation and work authorization.
10 U.S. Congress, Senate, *Health Equity and Access under the Law for Immigrant Families (HEAL ACT) Act of 2021*, S 1660, 117th Cong., 1st sess., introduced in Senate May 17, 2021. See www.congress.gov.
11 U.S. Congress, House, *Lifting Immigrant Families Through Benefits Access Restoration (LIFT the BAR ACT) Act of 2021*, HR 5227, 117th Cong., 1st sess., introduced in House September 10, 2021. See www.congress.gov.
12 See Kaiser Family Foundation 2022.
13 Ibid.
14 Kaiser Family Foundation, www.kff.org.
15 Blumenthal et al. 2020.
16 Wells 2021.
17 Blumenthal et al. 2020; Bassett, Chen, and Krieger 2020; Millett et al. 2020; Alan Nelson 2002; Raifman and Raifman 2020.
18 Blumenthal et al. 2020.
19 June 13, 2022. See Johns Hopkins University COVID-19 Dashboard: https://coronavirus.jhu.edu.
20 Blumenthal et al. 2020; Ramgobin et al. 2021.
21 Parker, Igielnik, and Kochhar 2021.
22 Igra et al. 2021.
23 Palosky 2022.
24 Amankwah-Amoah 2022; Plott, Kachalia, and Sharfstein 2020.
25 Sirleaf 2021.
26 Jakubiec 2022; King et al. 2023.
27 Glied and Altman 2017.

28 See Arendt 2005.
29 See Kleinman 2020.
30 Coutin 2000; De Genova 2002; 2004; 2013; Donato and Armenta 2011; Menjívar and Abrego 2012.
31 Kaur et al. 2021.
32 Nguyen-Ngo 2020; Salinas and Salinas 2022.
33 Hoekstra 2021; Jimenez 2021; Marrow and Joseph 2015; Park 2011; Park, Jimenez, and Hoekstra 2017.
34 Pew Research Center Poll (Jones 2020).
35 C. J. L. Murray and Frenk 2010; Reinhardt, Hussey, and Anderson 2004; Ridic, Gleason, and Ridic 2012; Schneider and Squires 2017.
36 Ridic, Gleason, and Ridic 2012.
37 Galvani et al. 2022.
38 Ibid.
39 Johnson, Kishore, and Berwick 2020.
40 Ibid.
41 Ibid., 134.
42 Park, Jimenez, and Hoekstra 2017.

BIBLIOGRAPHY

Abel, Emily. 2011. "Patient Dumping in New York City, 1877–1917." *American Journal of Public Health* 101 (5): 789–795.

Ackerman, Todd. 2011. "Still No Solution for Illegal Immigrants' Long-Term Care Costs." *Houston Chronicle*, October 30, 2011.

Adebowale, Victor, and Mala Rao. 2020. "Racism in Medicine: Why Equality Matters to Everyone." *BMJ* 368 (m530).

Aderath, Maya. 2020. "The United States Has a Long History of Mutual Aid Organizing." *Jacobin*, June 14, 2020. https://jacobin.com.

Adhikari, Samrachana, Nicholas P. Pantaleo, Justin M. Feldman, Olugbenga Ogedegbe, Lorna Thorpe, and Andrea B. Troxel. 2020. "Assessment of Community-Level Disparities in Coronavirus Disease 2019 (COVID-19) Infections and Deaths in Large US Metropolitan Areas." *JAMA Network Open* 3 (7), July 28, 2020.

Aguirre, Adalberto. 2012. "Arizona's SB1070, Latino Immigrants and the Framing of Anti-Immigrant Policies." *Latino Studies* 10 (3): 385–394.

Alltucker, Ken. 2015. "New Arizona Law Puts Subsidized Health Insurance at Risk." *AZ Central*, April 15, 2015. www.azcentral.com.

Amankwah-Amoah, Joseph. 2022. "COVID-19 and Counterfeit Vaccines: Global Implications, New Challenges and Opportunities." *Health Policy and Technology* 11 (2): 100630.

Anand, Nikhil. 2017. *Hydraulic City: Water and the Infrastructures of Citizenship in Mumbai*. Durham, NC: Duke University Press.

Andrulis, Dennis P., and Nadia J. Siddiqui. 2011. "Health Reform Holds Both Risks and Rewards for Safety-Net Providers and Racially and Ethnically Diverse Patients." *Health Affairs* 30 (10): 1830–1836.

Ansell, David A., and Robert L. Schiff. 1987. "Patient Dumping: Status, Implications, and Policy Recommendations." *JAMA* 257 (11): 1500–1502.

Appel, Hannah, Nikhil Anand, and Akhil Gupta. 2018. "Introduction: Temporality, Politics, and the Promise of Infrastructure." In *The Promise of Infrastructure*, edited by Hannah Appel, Nikhil Anand, and Akhil Gupta, 1–40. Durham, NC: Duke University Press.

Aptekar, Sofya. 2020. "Doctors as Migration Brokers in the Mandatory Medical Screenings of Immigrants to the United States." *Journal of Ethnic and Migration Studies* 46 (9): 1865–1885.

Arendt, Hannah. 2005. *Responsibility and Judgment*. New York: Schocken Books.

Arnold, Amanda. 2020. "So You Want to Get Involved in Mutual Aid." *The Cut,* September 30, 2020. www.thecut.com.

Artiga, Samantha, Nambi Ndugga, and Olivia Pham. 2021. "Immigrant Access to COVID-19 Vaccines: Key Issues to Consider." Henry J. Kaiser Family Foundation, January 13, 2021. www.kff.org.

Asad, Asad L. 2020. "On the Radar: System Embeddedness and Latin American Immigrants' Perceived Risk of Deportation." *Law & Society Review* 54 (1): 133–167.

Associated Press. 2012. "Finger-Wagging Arizona Governor Says Obama Was the Disrespectful One." *Mercury News,* January 26, 2012.

Bacong, Adrian Matias, and Cecilia Menjívar. 2021. "Recasting the Immigrant Health Paradox Through Intersections of Legal Status and Race." *Journal of Immigrant and Minority Health* 23 (5): 1092–1104.

Barnett, Jessica C., and Edward R. Berchick. 2017. "Health Insurance Coverage in the United States: 2016." Current Population Reports, P60–260. Washington, DC: US Government Printing Office.

Bassett, Mary T. 2016. "Beyond Berets: The Black Panthers as Health Activists." *American Journal of Public Health* 106 (10): 1741–1743.

———. 2019. "No Justice, No Health: The Black Panther Party's Fight for Health in Boston and beyond." *Journal of African American Studies* 23 (4): 352–363.

Bassett, Mary T., Jarvis T. Chen, and Nancy Krieger. 2020. "Variation in Racial/Ethnic Disparities in COVID-19 Mortality by Age in the United States: A Cross-Sectional Study." *PLoS Medicine* 17 (10): e1003402.

Baxter, Kevin. 2014. "Arizona Gov. Jan Brewer Dealt Legal Blow over Medicaid Expansion Plan." *Los Angeles Times,* December 31, 2014.

Baynton, Douglas C. 2005. "Defectives in the Land: Disability and American Immigration Policy, 1882–1924." *Journal of American Ethnic History* 24 (3): 31–44.

Becerra, David. 2016. "Anti-Immigration Policies and Fear of Deportation: A Human Rights Issue." *Journal of Human Rights and Social Work* 1 (3): 109–119.

Beitler, Jeremy R., Aaron M. Mittel, Richard Kallet, Robert Kacmarek, Dean Hess, Richard Branson, Murray Olson, Ivan Garcia, Barbara Powell, and David S. Wang. 2020. "Ventilator Sharing during an Acute Shortage Caused by the COVID-19 Pandemic." *American Journal of Respiratory and Critical Care Medicine* 202 (4): 600–604.

Belabas, Warda, and Lasse Gerrits. 2017. "Going the Extra Mile? How Street-Level Bureaucrats Deal with the Integration of Immigrants." *Social Policy & Administration* 51 (1): 133–150.

Berchick, Edward, Jessica Barnett, and Rachel Upton. 2019. "Health Insurance Coverage in the United States: 2018." Washington, DC: US Government Printing Office.

Berk, Marc L., and Claudia L. Schur. 2001. "The Effect of Fear on Access to Care among Undocumented Latino Immigrants." *Journal of Immigrant Health* 3 (3): 151–156.

Bernstein, Hamutal, Jorge Gonzale, Dulce Gonzalez, and Jahnavi Jagannath. 2020. "Immigrant-Serving Organizations' Perspectives on the COVID-19 Crisis." Urban Institute. www.urban.org.

Beyer, Scott. 2015. "The Texas Medical Center: Houston's Medical Mini-City." *Forbes*, December 11, 2015. www.forbes.com.

Blumenthal, David, Elizabeth J. Fowler, Melinda Abrams, and Sara R. Collins. 2020. "Covid-19—Implications for the Health Care System." *New England Journal of Medicine* 383: 1483–1488.

Boehrer, Fred. 2003. "Anarchism and Downward Mobility: Is Finishing Last the Least We Can Do?" *Contemporary Justice Review* 6 (1): 37–45.

Bonilla-Silva, Eduardo. 2020. "Color-Blind Racism in Pandemic Times." *Sociology of Race and Ethnicity* 8 (3): 343–354.

Borrelli, Lisa Marie. 2019. "The Border inside–Organizational Socialization of Street-Level Bureaucrats in the European Migration Regime." *Journal of Borderlands Studies* 36 (4): 1–20.

Bourdieu, Pierre. 1991. *Language and Symbolic Power*. Cambridge, MA: Harvard University Press.

Bradley, Ryan, Joanna Harnett, Kieran Cooley, Erica McIntyre, Joshua Goldenberg, and Jon Adams. 2019. "Naturopathy as a Model of Prevention-Oriented, Patient-Centered Primary Care: A Disruptive Innovation in Health Care." *Medicina* 55 (9): 603.

Braun, Virginia, and Victoria Clarke. 2006. "Using Thematic Analysis in Psychology." *Qualitative Research in Psychology* 3 (2): 77–101.

Braveman, Paula A., Shiriki Kumanyika, Jonathan Fielding, Thomas LaVeist, Luisa N. Borrell, Ron Manderscheid, and Adewale Troutman. 2011. "Health Disparities and Health Equity: The Issue Is Justice." *American Journal of Public Health* 101 (S1): S149–S155.

Brill, Steven. 2015. *America's Bitter Pill: Money, Politics, Backroom Deals, and the Fight to Fix Our Broken Healthcare System*. New York: Random House.

Brown, Henry S., Kimberly J. Wilson, and Jacqueline L. Angel. 2015. "Mexican Immigrant Health: Health Insurance Coverage Implications." *Journal of Health Care for the Poor and Underserved* 26 (3): 990–1004.

Brown, Phil, Stephen Zavestoski, Sabrina McCormick, Brian Mayer, Rachel Morello-Frosch, and Rebecca Gasior Altman. 2004. "Embodied Health Movements: New Approaches to Social Movements in Health." *Sociology of Health & Illness* 26 (1): 50–80.

Bryson, John R., Mark McGuiness, and Robert G. Ford. 2002. "Chasing a 'Loose and Baggy Monster': Almshouses and the Geography of Charity." *Area* 34 (1): 48–58.

Burt, Ronald S. 2000. "The Network Structure of Social Capital." *Research in Organizational Behavior* 22: 345–423.

———. 2004. "Structural Holes and Good Ideas." *American Journal of Sociology* 110 (2): 349–399.

———. 2005. *Brokerage and Closure: An Introduction to Social Capital*. New York: Oxford University Press.

California State Auditor. 1999. "Department of Health Services: Use of Its Port of Entry Fraud Detection Program Is No Longer Justified." Bureau of State Audits. www.bsa.ca.gov.

Campbell, Andrea Louise, and Lara Shore-Sheppard. 2020. "The Social, Political, and Economic Effects of the Affordable Care Act: Introduction to the Issue." *RSF: The Russell Sage Foundation Journal of the Social Sciences* 6 (2): 1–40.

Campbell, Kristina M. 2011. "The Road to SB 1070: How Arizona Became Ground Zero for the Immigrants' Rights Movement and the Continuing Struggle for Latino Civil Rights in America." *Harvard Latino Law Review* 14: 1.

Carse, Ashley. 2016. "Keyword: Infrastructure: How a Humble French Engineering Term Shaped the Modern World." In *Infrastructures and Social Complexity: A Companion*, edited by Penny Harvey, Casper Bruun Jensen, and Atsuro Morita, 27–39. New York: Routledge.

Castañeda, Heide, Seth M. Holmes, Daniel S. Madrigal, Maria-Elena DeTrinidad Young, Naomi Beyeler, and James Quesada. 2015. "Immigration as a Social Determinant of Health." *Annual Review of Public Health* 36: 375–392.

Catholic Worker Movement. 2023. "Search CW Communities." www.catholicworker.org.

Cervantes, Andrea Gómez, and Cecilia Menjívar. 2020. "Legal Violence, Health and Access to Care: Latina Immigrants in Rural and Urban Kansas." *Journal of Health and Social Behavior* 61 (3): 1–17.

Chen, Mel. 2020. "Feminisms in the Air." *Signs* 47 (1): 22–29.

Cheney, Kyle, and Jason Millman. 2013. "Brewer Wins Medicaid Expansion." *Politico*, June 13, 2013. www.politico.com.

Chomsky, Noam. 1999. *Profit over People: Neoliberalism and Global Order*. New York: Seven Stories Press.

Christopher, Andrea S., and Dominic Caruso. 2015. "Promoting Health as a Human Right in the Post-ACA United States." *AMA Journal of Ethics* 17 (10): 958–965.

Clare, Eli. 1999. *Exile and Pride: Disability, Queerness and Liberation*. Cambridge, MA: South End Press.

Collins, Patricia Hill. 2008. *Black Feminist Thought: Knowledge, Consciousness, and the Politics of Empowerment*. New York: Routledge.

Congressional Research Service. 2021. "Medicaid Disproportionate Share Hospital (DSH) Reductions." Congressional Research Service. http://crsreports.congress.gov.

Coughlin, Teresa A., Sharon K. Long, Edward Sheen, and Jennifer Tolbert. 2012. "How Five Leading Safety-Net Hospitals Are Preparing for the Challenges and Opportunities of Health Care Reform." *Health Affairs* 31 (8): 1690–1697.

Coutin, Susan Bibler. 2000. *Legalizing Moves: Salvadoran Immigrants' Struggle for U.S. Residency*. Ann Arbor: University of Michigan Press.

Cox, Cynthia, Michelle Long, Ashley Semanskee, Rabah Kamal, Gary Claxton, and Larry Levitt. 2016. "2017 Premium Changes and Insurer Participation in the Affordable Care Act's Health Insurance Marketplaces." www.kff.org.

Coy, Patrick G. 2001. "An Experiment in Personalist Politics: The Catholic Worker Movement and Nonviolent Action." *Peace & Change* 26 (1): 78–94.

Crow, Liz. 1996. "Including All of Our Lives: Renewing the Social Model of Disability." In *Encounters with Strangers: Feminism and Disability*. London: The Women's Press Ltd.

D'Agostini, Gabriella M. 2019. "Treading on Sacred Land: First Amendment Implications of ICE's Targeting of Churches." *Michigan Law Review* 118: 315.

Darnell, Julie S. 2010. "Free Clinics in the United States: A Nationwide Survey." *Archives of Internal Medicine* 170 (11): 946–953.

Day, Dorothy. 1952. *The Long Loneliness*. San Francisco: Harper & Row.

De Genova, Nicholas. 2002. "Migrant 'Illegality' and Deportability in Everyday Life." *Annual Review of Anthropology* 31: 419–447.

———. 2004. "The Legal Production of Mexican/Migrant 'Illegality'." *Latino Studies* 2: 160–85.

———. 2013. "Spectacles of Migrant 'Illegality': The Scene of Exclusion, the Obscene of Inclusion." *Ethnic and Racial Studies* 36 (7): 1180–1198.

Deines, Helen. 2008. "The Catholic Worker Movement: Communities of Personal Hospitality and Justice." *Social Work and Christianity* 35 (4): 429.

DeVoe, Jennifer. 2008. "The Unsustainable US Health Care System: A Blueprint for Change." *Annals of Family Medicine* 6 (3): 263–266.

Donato, Katharine M., and Amada Armenta. 2011. "What We Know about Unauthorized Migration." *Annual Review of Sociology* 37: 529–543.

Ebert, Kim, Wenjie Liao, and Emily P. Estrada. 2020. "Apathy and Color-Blindness in Privatized Immigration Control." *Sociology of Race and Ethnicity* 6 (4): 533–547.

Edlins, Mariglynn, and Jennica Larrison. 2020. "Street-Level Bureaucrats and the Governance of Unaccompanied Migrant Children." *Public Policy and Administration* 35 (4): 403–423.

Elder, Charles R. 2013. "Integrating Naturopathy: Can We Move Forward?" *Permanente Journal* 17 (4): 80.

Enfield, Lisa M., and David P. Sklar. 1988. "Patient Dumping in the Hospital Emergency Department: Renewed Interest in an Old Problem." *American Journal of Law & Medicine* 13 (4): 561–595.

Espiritu, Yén Le, and Lan Duong. 2022. *Departures: An Introduction to Critical Refugee Studies*. Berkeley: University of California Press.

Estrada, Emily P., Kim Ebert, and Wenjie Liao. 2020. "Polarized toward Apathy: An Analysis of the Privatized Immigration-Control Debate in the Trump Era." *PS: Political Science & Politics* 53 (4): 679–684.

Evans, Patricia R. 1987. "'Likely to Become a Public Charge': Immigration in the Backwaters of Administrative Law, 1882–1933." PhD diss., George Washington University.

Evashwick, Connie. 1989. "Creating the Continuum of Care." *Health Matrix* 7 (1): 30–39.

Fairchild, Amy. 2005. "Comment: Historicizing the Notion of Disability." *Journal of American Ethnic History* 24 (3): 45–48.

Families USA. 2017. "In Their Own Words: Republican Governors Support Medicaid Expansion." www.familiesusa.org.

Farmer, Paul. 2004. "An Anthropology of Structural Violence." *Current Anthropology* 45 (3): 305–325.

Feder, Judith, Harriet L. Komisar, and Marlene Niefeld. 2000. "Long-Term Care in the United States: An Overview." *Health Affairs* 19 (3): 40–56.

Felland, Laurie, Peter J. Cunningham, Annie Doubleday, and Cannon Warren. 2016. *Effects of the Affordable Care Act on Safety Net Hospitals.* Washington, DC: Mathematica Policy Research.

Fernandez, Roberto M., and Roger V. Gould. 1994. "A Dilemma of State Power: Brokerage and Influence in the National Health Policy Domain." *American Journal of Sociology* 99 (6): 1455–1491.

Fields, Desiree J., and Stuart N. Hodkinson. 2018. "Housing Policy in Crisis: An International Perspective." *Housing Policy Debate* 28 (1): 1–5.

Finegold, Kenneth, Ann Conmy, Rose C. Chu, Arielle Bosworth, and Benjamin D. Sommers. 2021. "Trends in the U.S. Uninsured Population, 2010–2020." Issue Brief. ASPE Office of Health Policy.

Forman, Tyrone A. 2004. "Color-Blind Racism and Racial Indifference: The Role of Racial Apathy in Facilitating Enduring Inequalities." In *The Changing Terrain of Race and Ethnicity,* edited by Maria Krysan and Amanda E. Lewis, 43–66. New York: The Russell Sage Foundation.

Forman, Tyrone A., and Amanda E. Lewis. 2006. "Racial Apathy and Hurricane Katrina: The Social Anatomy of Prejudice in the Post-Civil Rights Era." *Du Bois Review: Social Science Research on Race* 3 (1): 175–202.

Foucault, Michel. 1975. *The Birth of the Clinic: An Archaeology of Medical Perception.* New York: Vintage Books.

Frierson, Jannie C. 2020. "The Black Panther Party and the Fight for Health Equity." *Journal of Health Care for the Poor and Underserved* 31 (4): 1520–1529.

Galvani, Alison P., Alyssa S. Parpia, Abhishek Pandey, Pratha Sah, Kenneth Colón, Gerald Friedman, Travis Campbell, James G. Kahn, Burton H. Singer, and Meagan C. Fitzpatrick. 2022. "Universal Healthcare as Pandemic Preparedness: The Lives and Costs That Could Have Been Saved during the COVID-19 Pandemic." *Proceedings of the National Academy of Sciences* 119 (25): e2200536119.

Gammage, Jennifer. 2021. "Solidarity, Not Charity: Mutual Aid's An-Archic History." *Blog of the American Philosophical Association.* January 25, 2021. https://blog .apaonline.org.

Garcés, Isabel C., Isabel C. Scarinci, and Lynda Harrison. 2006. "An Examination of Sociocultural Factors Associated with Health and Health Care Seeking among Latina Immigrants." *Journal of Immigrant and Minority Health* 8 (4): 377–385.

Gardner, Martha. 2009. *The Qualities of a Citizen: Women, Immigration, and Citizenship, 1870–1965.* Princeton, NJ: Princeton University Press.

Garfield, Rachel, Kendal Orgera, and Anthony Damico. 2021. "The Coverage Gap: Uninsured Poor Adults in States that Do Not Expand Medicaid." Henry J. Kaiser Family Foundation. www.kff.org.

Gee, Gilbert C., Anna Hing, Selina Mohammed, Derrick C. Tabor, and David R. Williams. 2019. "Racism and the Life Course: Taking Time Seriously." *American Journal of Public Health* 109 (S1): s43–s47.

Genworth. 2020. "Cost of Long Term Care by State | Cost of Care Report." 2020. www.genworth.com.

Geyman, John. 2021. "COVID-19 Has Revealed America's Broken Health Care System: What Can We Learn?" *International Journal of Health Services* 51 (2): 188–194.

Glied, Sherry A., and Stuart H. Altman. 2017. "Beyond Antitrust: Health Care and Health Insurance Market Trends and the Future of Competition." *Health Affairs* 36 (9): 1572–1577.

Golash-Boza, Tanya. 2009. "The Immigration Industrial Complex: Why We Enforce Immigration Policies Destined to Fail." *Sociology Compass* 3 (2): 295–309.

Goldman, Dana P., James P. Smith, and Neeraj Sood. 2006. "Immigrants and the Cost of Medical Care." *Health Affairs* 25 (6): 1700–1711.

Gordon, Todd. 2005. "The Political Economy of Law-and-Order Policies: Policing, Class Struggle, and Neoliberal Restructuring." *Studies in Political Economy* 75 (1): 53–77.

Gould, Roger V., and Roberto M. Fernandez. 1989. "Structures of Mediation: A Formal Approach to Brokerage in Transaction Networks." *Sociological Methodology* 19, 89–126.

Grouse, Lawrence. 2014. "Cost-Effective Medicine vs. the Medical-Industrial Complex." *Journal of Thoracic Disease* 6 (9): 203–206.

Hacker, Karen, Jocelyn Chu, Lisa Arsenault, and Robert P. Marlin. 2012. "Provider's Perspectives on the Impact of Immigration and Customs Enforcement (ICE) Activity on Immigrant Health." *Journal of Health Care for the Poor and Underserved* 23 (2): 651–665.

Harris County Healthcare Alliance. 2016. *The State of Health: Houston & Harris County 2015–2016*. Harris County Healthcare Alliance. www.houstonstateofhealth .com.

Harris Health System. 2000. "Harris County Hospital District Financial Assistance Program." Harris Health System. www.harrishealth.org.

———. 2018. "Harris Health: About Us." Harris Health System. www.harrishealth.org.

———. 2020. "Patient Eligibility." Harris Health System. www.harrishealth.org.

Harvey, David. 2020. "Anti-Capitalist Politics in the Time of COVID-19." *Jacobin*, March 20, 2020. https://jacobinmag.com.

Hauslohner, Abigail, and Janell Ross. 2017. "Trump Administration Circulates More Draft Immigration Restrictions, Focusing on Protecting U.S. Jobs." *Washington Post*, January 31, 2017.

HealthCare.Gov. 2022. "No Health Insurance." HealthCare.Gov. www.healthcare.gov.

Henderson, Michael, and D. Sunshine Hillygus. 2011. "The Dynamics of Health Care Opinion, 2008–2010: Partisanship, Self-Interest, and Racial Resentment." *Journal of Health Politics, Policy and Law* 36 (6): 945–960.

Heyman, Josiah McC., Guillermina Gina Núñez, and Victor Talavera. 2009. "Health-care Access and Barriers for Unauthorized Immigrants in El Paso County, Texas." *Family & Community Health* 32 (1): 4–21.

Higham, John. 1976. "Politics of Immigration Restriction." *Immigration & Nationality Law Review* 1 (1).

Himmelstein, David U., Steffie Woolhandler, Martha Harnly, Michael B. Bader, Ralph Silber, Howard D. Backer, and Alice A. Jones. 1984. "Patient Transfers: Medical Practice as Social Triage." *American Journal of Public Health* 74 (5): 494–497.

Hoekstra, Erin. 2021. "'Not a Free Version of a Broken System:' Medical Humanitarian-ism and Immigrant Health Justice in the United States." *Social Science & Medicine* 285: 114287.

Hoekstra, Erin, and Anthony M. Jimenez. 2023. "Versatile Brokerage: Migrant-Provider Relationships in the Third Net of the US Healthcare System." *Journal of Ethnic and Migration Studies*, 1–20.

Holmes, Seth M. 2011. "Structural Vulnerability and Hierarchies of Ethnicity and Citizenship on the Farm." *Medical Anthropology* 30 (4): 425–449.

———. 2012. "The Clinical Gaze in the Practice of Migrant Health: Mexican Immigrants in the United States." *Social Science & Medicine* 74 (6): 873–881.

Howland, Rebecca, Vishaal Pegany, Carolina Coleman, and John Connolly. 2014. "Remaining Uninsured: A Population Profile." Insure the Uninsured Project. http://itup.org.

Hutchinson, Edward P. 1987. *Legislative History of American Immigration Policy, 1798–1965*. Philadelphia: University of Pennsylvania Press.

Igra, Mark, Nora Kenworthy, Cadence Luchsinger, and Jin-Kyu Jung. 2021. "Crowd-funding as a Response to COVID-19: Increasing Inequities at a Time of Crisis." *Social Science & Medicine* 282: 114105.

Immigrant Legal Resource Center. 2022. "An Overview of Public Charge." May 4, 2022. www.ilrc.org.

Islam, Nadia, and Naheed Ahmed. 2021. "Anti-Immigrant Rhetoric and Policy as Manifestations of Structural Racism—Implications for Advancing Health Equity." *JAMA Network Open* 4 (7): e2118299.

Islam, Nadia, Smiti Kapadia Nadkarni, Deborah Zahn, Megan Skillman, Simona C. Kwon, and Chau Trinh-Shevrin. 2015. "Integrating Community Health Workers within Patient Protection and Affordable Care Act Implementation." *Journal of Public Health Management and Practice* 21 (1): 42.

Jahnke, Lauren, Nadia Siddiqui, Dennis Andrulis, and Swapna Reddy. 2015. "Snapshot of Medicaid 1115 Waiver and Other State-Based Delivery System Transformations." Texas Health Institute. www.texashealthinstitute.org.

Jakubiec, Pauline. 2022. "Yea or Nay? Hospital Mergers and Acquisitions." *Journal of Health Care Finance* 48 (2).

Jimenez, Anthony M. 2021. "The Legal Violence of Care: Navigating the US Health Care System While Undocumented and Illegible." *Social Science & Medicine*.

——. 2022. "'All Are Deserving': Racialized Conditions of Immigrant Deserving-ness in a Catholic Worker Movement-Inspired Non-Governmental Organization." *American Behavioral Scientist* 66 (13): 1758–1776.

Jimenez, Anthony M., and Timothy W. Collins. 2017. "'How Do We Not Go Back to the Factor?' Symbolic Violence within Neoliberal Urban Development for a Latina-Led NGO." *City* 21 (6): 737–753.

Johnson, Micah, Sanjay Kishore, and Donald M. Berwick. 2020. "Medicare for All: An Analysis of Key Policy Issues: A Discussion of Design Issues and Options Raised by Pending Medicare for All Legislation and Proposals." *Health Affairs* 39 (1): 133–141.

Jones, Bradley. 2020. "Increasing Share of Americans Favor a Single Government Pro-gram to Provide Health Care Coverage." Pew Research Center. www.pewresearch .org.

Joseph, Tiffany D. 2017. "Falling through the Coverage Cracks: How Documentation Status Minimizes Immigrants' Access to Health Care." *Journal of Health Politics, Policy and Law* 42 (5): 961–984.

Kaiser Commission on Key Facts. 2013. "Key Facts on Health Coverage for Low-Income Immigrants Today and Under the Affordable Care Act." Henry J. Kaiser Family Foundation. www.kff.org.

Kaur, Harneel, Ammar Saad, Olivia Magwood, Qasem Alkhateeb, Christine Mathew, Gina Khalaf, and Kevin Pottie. 2021. "Understanding the Health and Housing Expe-riences of Refugees and Other Migrant Populations Experiencing Homelessness or Vulnerable Housing: A Systematic Review Using GRADE-CERQual." *Canadian Medical Association Open Access Journal* 9 (2): E681–E692.

Kawachi, Ichiro, and Bruce P. Kennedy. 1997. "Socioeconomic Determinants of Health: Health and Social Cohesion: Why Care about Income Inequality?" *BMJ* 314 (7086): 1037.

——. 1999. "Income Inequality and Health: Pathways and Mechanisms." *Health Ser-vices Research* 34: 215–227.

Kaye, H. Stephen, Charlene Harrington, and Mitchell P. LaPlante. 2010. "Long-Term Care: Who Gets It, Who Provides It, Who Pays, and How Much?" *Health Affairs* 29 (1): 11–21.

Kaye, H. Stephen, Mitchell P. LaPlante, and Charlene Harrington. 2009. "Do Noninsti-tutional Long-Term Care Services Reduce Medicaid Spending?" *Health Affairs* 28 (1): 262–272.

Kellermann, Arthur L., and Bela B. Hackman. 1988. "Emergency Department Patient 'Dumping': An Analysis of Interhospital Transfers to the Regional Medical Center at Memphis, Tennessee." *American Journal of Public Health* 78 (10): 1287–1292.

Kelley, A. Taylor, and Renuka Tipirneni. 2018. "Care for Undocumented Immigrants—Rethinking State Flexibility in Medicaid Waivers." *New England Journal of Medicine* 378 (18): 1661–1663.

Kelly, Marisa. 1994. "Theories of Justice and Street-Level Discretion." *Journal of Public Administration Research and Theory* 4 (2): 119–140.

Kemble, Sarah. 2000. "Charity Care Programs: Part of the Solution or Part of the Problem?" *Public Health Reports* 115 (5): 419.

Kennedy, Edward H., M. Todd Greene, and Sanjay Saint. 2013. "Estimating Hospital Costs of Catheter-Associated Urinary Tract Infection." *Journal of Hospital Medicine* 8 (9): 519–522.

King, Jaime S., Alexandra D. Montague, Daniel Arnold, and Thomas L. Greaney. 2023. "Antitrust's Healthcare Conundrum: Cross-Market Mergers and the Rise of System Power." *Hastings Law Journal* 74 (4): 1057–1120.

Kleinman, Arthur. 2020. *The Illness Narratives: Suffering, Healing, and the Human Condition.* New York: Basic Books.

Kline, Nolan. 2017. "Pathogenic Policy: Immigrant Policing, Fear, and Parallel Medical Systems in the US South." *Medical Anthropology* 35 (4): 396–420.

———. 2019. *Pathogenic Policing: Immigration Enforcement and Health in the US South.* New Brunswick, NJ: Rutgers University Press.

Klineberg, Stephen, Jie Wu, Kiara Douds, and Diana Ramirez. 2014. "Shared Prospects: Hispanics and the Future of Houston." Rice University Kinder Institute for Urban Research. Houston: Rice University.

Koetting, Michael J. 1989. "Correctly Defining and Assessing the Causes of Hospital Dumping." *American Journal of Public Health* 79 (6): 780.

Komisar, Harriet L., and Marlene Niefeld. 2000. "Long-Term Care Needs, Care Arrangements, and Unmet Needs among Community Adults: Findings from the National Health Interview Survey on Disability." Working Paper no. IWP-00-102. Institute for Health Care Research and Policy, Georgetown University.

Kovic, Christine. 2014. "Demanding to Be Seen and Heard: Latino Immigrant Organizing and the Defense of Human Rights in Houston." *City & Society* 26 (1): 10–28.

Krieger, Nancy. 1994. "Epidemiology and the Web of Causation: Has Anyone Seen the Spider?" *Social Science and Medicine* 39 (7): 887–903.

———. 2001. "Theories for Social Epidemiology in the Twenty-First Century: An Ecosocial Perspective." *International Journal of Epidemiology* 30 (4): 668–677.

Ku, Leighton, and Brian Bruen. 2013. "The Use of Public Assistance Benefits by Citizens and Non-Citizen Immigrants in the United States." Cato Working Paper. Cato Institute. www.cato.org.

Kwok, Abe. 2020. "What to Know about the Maricopa County Special Health Care District Election." *AZ Central*, July 14, 2020. www.azcentral.com.

Lakoff, Andrew. 2020. "'The Supply Chain Must Continue': Becoming Essential in the Pandemic Emergency." *Items*, November 5, 2020. https://items.ssrc.org.

Lamphere, Louise. 2005. "Providers and Staff Respond to Medicaid Managed Care: The Unintended Consequences of Reform in New Mexico." *Medical Anthropology Quarterly* 19 (1): 3–25.

Levine, Carol, Deborah Halper, Ariella Peist, and David A. Gould. 2010. "Bridging Troubled Waters: Family Caregivers, Transitions, and Long-Term Care." *Health Affairs* 29 (1): 116–124.

Levy, Helen, Andrew Ying, and Nicholas Bagley. 2020. "What's Left of the Affordable Care Act? A Progress Report." *RSF: The Russell Sage Foundation Journal of the Social Sciences* 6 (2): 42–66.

Lewin, Marion Ein, and Stuart Altman, eds. 2000. *America's Health Care Safety Net: Intact but Endangered.* Washington, DC: National Academies Press.

Lipsky, Michael. 1980. *Street-Level Bureaucracy: Dilemmas of the Individual in Public Service.* New York: Russell Sage Foundation.

———. 2010. *Street-Level Bureaucracy: Dilemmas of the Individual in Public Service.* New York: Russell Sage Foundation.

List, Justin M. 2011. "Beyond Charity: Social Justice and Health Care." *AMA Journal of Ethics* 13 (8): 565–568.

López-Sanders, Laura. 2017a. "Changing the Navigator's Course: How the Increasing Rationalization of Healthcare Influences Access for Undocumented Immigrants under the Affordable Care Act." *Social Science & Medicine* 178: 46–54.

———. 2017b. "Navigating Health Care: Brokerage and Access for Undocumented Latino Immigrants under the 2010 Affordable Care Act." *Journal of Ethnic and Migration Studies* 43 (12): 2072–2088.

MacKenzie, Thomas D., Teresa Kukolja, Robert House, Amanda A. Loehr, Joel M. Hirsh, and Kathy A. Boyle. 2012. "A Discharge Panel at Denver Health, Focused on Complex Patients, May Have Influenced Decline in Length-of-Stay." *Health Affairs* 31 (8): 1786–1795.

Magaña, Lisa, and Erik Lee, eds. 2013. *Latino Politics and Arizona's Immigration Law SB 1070.* New York: Springer.

Maldonado, Angeles. 2013. "Raids, Race, and Lessons of Fear and Resistance: Narratives and Discourse in the Immigration Movement in Arizona." PhD diss., Arizona State University.

Maldonado, Cynthia Z., Robert M. Rodriguez, Jesus R. Torres, Yvette S. Flores, and Luis M. Lovato. 2013. "Fear of Discovery among Latino Immigrants Presenting to the Emergency Department." *Academic Emergency Medicine* 20 (2): 155–161.

Maniscalco, Sebastian. 2020. *Doorbell (What's Wrong with People?).* Video, 4:51. www.youtube.com/watch?v=5CznoAW2k1I.

Marmot, Michael. 2021. "Social Justice, Human Rights and Health Equity." *Journal of Public Health* 43 (3): e423–e424.

Marrow, Helen B., and Tiffany D. Joseph. 2015. "Excluded and Frozen Out: Unauthorised Immigrants' (Non)Access to Care after US Health Care Reform." *Journal of Ethnic and Migration Studies* 41 (14): 2253–2273.

Marsden, Peter. 1982. "Brokerage Behavior in Restricted Exchange Networks." *Social Structure and Network Analysis* 7 (4): 341–410.

Maynard-Moody, Steven, and Michael Musheno. 2000. "State Agent or Citizen Agent: Two Narratives of Discretion." *Journal of Public Administration Research and Theory* 10 (2): 329–358.

McDowell, Meghan G., and Nancy A. Wonders. 2009. "Keeping Migrants in Their Place: Technologies of Control and Racialized Public Space in Arizona." *Social Justice* 36 (2) (116): 54–72.

McKanan, Dan. 2008. *The Catholic Worker after Dorothy: Practicing the Works of Mercy in a New Generation.* Collegeville, MN: Liturgical Press.

McKay, Fiona H., and Ann R. Taket. 2020. *Health Equity, Social Justice, and Human Rights.* New York: Routledge.

Menjívar, Cecilia, and Leisy Abrego. 2012. "Legal Violence: Immigration Law and the Lives of Central American Immigrants." *American Journal of Sociology* 117 (5): 1380–1421.

Menjívar, Cecilia, W.P. Simmons, D. Alvord, and E.S. Valdez. 2018. "Immigration Enforcement, the Racialization of Legal Status, and Perceptions of the Police: Latinos in Chicago, Los Angeles, Houston, and Phoenix in Comparative Perspective." *Du Bois Review* 15 (1): 107–128.

Millett, Gregorio A., Austin T. Jones, David Benkeser, Stefan Baral, Laina Mercer, Chris Beyrer, Brian Honermann, et al. 2020. "Assessing Differential Impacts of COVID-19 on Black Communities." *Annals of Epidemiology* 47 (1): 37–44.

Minich, Julie Avril. 2016. "Enabling Whom? Critical Disability Studies Now." *Lateral* 5 (1).

Molloy, Luke J., Kim Walker, and Richard Lakeman. 2017. "Shared Worlds: Multi-Sited Ethnography and Nursing Research." *Nurse Researcher* 24 (4): 22–26.

Monday, Kimberly E., and Esmaeil Porsa. 2020. "Historic Times. Amazing People: 2020 Annual Report to the Community." Harris Health System. https://2020harrishealthannualreport.org.

Morse, Ann, Jeremy Meadows, Kirsten Rasmussen, and Sheri Steisel. 1998. *America's Newcomers: Mending the Safety Net for Immigrants.* Denver: National Conference of State Legislatures.

Morton, Keith, and John Saltmarsh. 1997. "Addams, Day, and Dewey: The Emergence of Community Service in American Culture." *Michigan Journal of Community Service Learning* 4 (1): 137–149.

Mueller, Jennifer. 2017. "Producing Colorblindness: Everyday Mechanisms of White Ignorance." *Social Problems* 64 (2): 219–238.

Mueller, Jennifer, and Rula Issa. 2016. "Consuming Black Pain: Reading Racial Ideology in Cultural Appetite for 12 Years a Slave." In *Race and Contention in Twenty-First Century U.S. Media*, edited by Jason A. Smith and Bhoomi K. Thakore, 131–147. New York: Routledge.

Muers, Rachel. 2021. "Always with You: Questioning the Theological Construction of the Un/Deserving Poor." *International Journal of Public Theology* 15 (1): 42–60.

Munson, Helen W. 1930. "The Care of the Sick in Almshouses." *American Journal of Nursing* 30 (1): 1226–1230.

Munson, Valerie J. 2017. "On Holy Ground: Church Sanctuary in the Trump Era." *Southwestern University Law Review* 47 (1): 49.

Murray, Christopher J.L., and Julio Frenk. 2010. "Ranking 37th—Measuring the Performance of the US Health Care System." *New England Journal of Medicine* 362 (2): 98–99.

Murray, Harry. 1990. *Do Not Neglect Hospitality.* Philadelphia, PA: Temple University Press.

National Humanities Center. 2009. *The Making of African American Identity—Volume I: 1500–1865.* http://nationalhumanitiescenter.org.

Navarro, Vicente. 2020. "The Consequences of Neoliberalism in the Current Pandemic." *International Journal of Health Services* 50 (3): 271–275.

Nelson, Alan. 2002. "Unequal Treatment: Confronting Racial and Ethnic Disparities in Health Care." *Journal of the National Medical Association* 94 (8): 666.

Nelson, Alondra. 2011. *Body and Soul: The Black Panther Party and the Fight against Medical Discrimination.* Minneapolis: University of Minnesota Press.

Nessel, Lori. 2012. "Disposable Workers: Applying a Human Rights Framework to Analyze Duties Owed to Seriously Injured or Ill Migrants." *Indiana Journal of Global Legal Studies* 19 (1): 61–103.

Nethercote, Megan. 2020. "Build-to-Rent and the Financialization of Rental Housing: Future Research Directions." *Housing Studies* 35 (5): 839–874.

New Hampshire Bureau of Labor. 1894. "Annual Report of the Bureau of Labor of the State of New Hampshire." Hathi Trust Digital Library. https://babel.hathitrust.org.

Nguyen-Ngo, Matt. 2020. "Addressing Labor Exploitation: An Examination of Undocumented Asian Americans in the Workplace." *Asian American Policy Review*, June 2. https://aapr.hkspublications.org.

Nibbe, Niki A. 2012. *Beyond the Free Clinics Origin Myth: Reconsidering Free Clinics in the Context of 1960s and 1970s Social Movements and Radical Health Activism.* MA thesis, University of California, San Francisco.

Niles, Meredith T., Farryl Bertmann, Emily H. Belarmino, Thomas Wentworth, Erin Biehl, and Roni Neff. 2020. "The Early Food Insecurity Impacts of COVID-19." *Nutrients* 12 (7): 2096.

Nill, Andrea Christina. 2011. "Latinos and SB 1070: Demonization, Dehumanization, and Disenfranchisement." *Harvard Latino Law Review* 14 (1): 35.

Norman, Jane. 2013. "Republican Governor of Arizona Says She'll Back Medicaid Expansion." *Commonwealth Fund*, January 13, 2013. www.commonwealthfund.org.

Norris, Louise. 2022. "Arizona and the ACA's Medicaid Expansion." HealthInsurance.org. Accessed May 10, 2023. www.healthinsurance.org.

Nutter, Donald O. 1987. "Medical Indigency and the Public Health Care Crisis." *New England Journal of Medicine* 316 (18): 1156–1158.

Okie, Susan. 2007. "Immigrants and Health Care-at the Intersection of Two Broken Systems." *New England Journal of Medicine* 357 (6): 525–529.

Ornelas, India J., Thespina J. Yamanis, and Raymond A. Ruiz. 2020. "The Health of Undocumented Latinx Immigrants: What We Know and Future Directions." *Annual Review of Public Health* 41: 289–308.

Page-Reeves, Janet, Joshua Niforatos, Shiraz Mishra, Lidia Regino, Andrew Gingrich, and Robert Bulten. 2013. "Health Disparity and Structural Violence: How Fear Undermines Health among Immigrants at Risk for Diabetes." *Journal of Health Disparities Research and Practice* 6 (2): 30.

Palosky, Craig. 2022. "1 in 10 Adults Owe Medical Debt, With Millions Owing More Than $10,000." Henry J. Kaiser Family Foundation. www.kff.org.

Park, Lisa Sun-Hee. 2005. *Consuming Citizenship: Children of Asian Immigrant Entrepreneurs.* Palo Alto: Stanford University Press.

———. 2011. *Entitled to Nothing: The Struggle for Immigrant Health Care in the Age of Welfare Reform.* New York: NYU Press.

———. 2018. "Medical Deportations: Blurring the Line Between Health Care and Immigration Enforcement." In *Immigration Policy in the Age of Punishment: Detention, Deportation and Border Control,* edited by David C. Brotherton and Philip Kretsedemas, 240–256. Columbia: Columbia University Press.

Park, Lisa Sun-Hee, Anthony Jimenez, and Erin Hoekstra. 2017. "Decolonizing the US Health Care System: Undocumented and Disabled after ACA." *Health Tomorrow: Interdisciplinarity and Internationality* 5 (1): 24–54.

Parker, Kim, Ruth Igielnik, and Rakesh Kochhar. 2021. "Unemployed Americans Are Feeling the Emotional Strain of Job Loss; Most Have Considered Changing Occupations." Pew Research Center. www.pewresearch.org.

Passel, Jeffrey S., and D'vera Cohn. 2016. "Size of U.S. Unauthorized Immigrant Workforce Stable After the Great Recession." Pew Research Center. www.pewhispanic.org.

Pellegrino, Edmund D. 1999. "The Commodification of Medical and Health Care: The Moral Consequences of a Paradigm Shift from a Professional to a Market Ethic." *Journal of Medicine and Philosophy* 24 (3): 243–266.

Phelan, Jo C., and Bruce G. Link. 2015. "Is Racism a Fundamental Cause of Inequalities in Health?" *Annual Review of Sociology* 41 (1): 311–330.

Phelan, Jo C., Bruce G. Link, and P. Tehranifar. 2010. "Social Conditions as Fundamental Causes of Health Inequalities: Theory, Evidence, and Policy Implications." *Journal of Health and Social Behavior* 51 (Suppl.): S28–S40.

Phillips, Marilyn, and Virginia Fitzsimons. 2015. "The Affordable Care Act: Impact on Case Managers." *Professional Case Management* 20 (6): 323–327.

Picarda, Hubert. 2014. *The Law and Practice Relating to Charities: First Supplement to the Fourth Edition,* Suppl. ed. Haywards Heath, UK: Bloomsbury Professional.

Piven, Frances Fox, and Richard A. Cloward. 1971. *Regulating the Poor: The Functions of Public Welfare.* New York: Pantheon Books.

Plott, Caroline F., Allen B. Kachalia, and Joshua M. Sharfstein. 2020. "Unexpected Health Insurance Profits and the COVID-19 Crisis." *JAMA* 324 (17): 1713–1714.

Portes, Alejandro, Patricia Fernández-Kelly, and Donald Light. 2012. "Life on the Edge: Immigrants Confront the American Health System." *Ethnic and Racial Studies* 35 (1): 3–22.

Portes, Alejandro, Donald Light, and Patricia Fernández-Kelly. 2009. "The U.S. Health System and Immigration: An Institutional Interpretation." *Sociological Forum* 24 (3): 487–514.

Portes, Alejandro, and Julia Sensenbrenner. 1993. "Embeddedness and Immigration: Notes on the Social Determinants of Economic Action." *American Journal of Sociology* 98 (6): 1320–1350.

Pullan, Brian. 2019. "Charity and Poor Relief: The Early Modern Period." Encyclopedia .com. Accessed May 11, 2023. www.encyclopedia.com.

Quesada, James, Laurie Kain Hart, and Philippe Bourgois. 2011. "Structural Vulnerability and Health: Latino Migrant Laborers in the United States." *Medical Anthropology* 30 (4): 339–362.

Raifman, Matthew A., and Julia R. Raifman. 2020. "Disparities in the Population at Risk of Severe Illness from COVID-19 by Race/Ethnicity and Income." *American Journal of Preventive Medicine* 59 (1): 137–139.

Ramgobin, Devyani, Brendan McClafferty, Courtney Kramer, Reshma Golamari, Brian McGillen, and Rohit Jain. 2021. "Papering over the Cracks: COVID-19's Amplification of the Failures of Employer-Based Health Insurance Coverage." *Journal of Community Hospital Internal Medicine Perspectives* 11 (1): 107–110.

Ramirez, Giorlando, Lucas Fox, Krutika Amin, and Cynthia Cox. 2021. "How ACA Marketplace Premiums Are Changing by County in 2022." Henry J. Kaiser Family Foundation. www.kff.org.

Ranney, Megan L., Valerie Griffeth, and Ashish K. Jha. 2020. "Critical Supply Shortages—the Need for Ventilators and Personal Protective Equipment during the Covid-19 Pandemic." *New England Journal of Medicine* 382 (18): e41.

Reinhardt, Uwe E., Peter S. Hussey, and Gerard F. Anderson. 2004. "US Health Care Spending in an International Context." *Health Affairs* 23 (3): 10–25.

Relman, Arnold S. 1980. "The New Medical-Industrial Complex." *New England Journal of Medicine* 303 (17): 963–970.

Rhodes, Scott D., Lilli Mann, Florence M. Simán, Eunyoung Song, Jorge Alonzo, Mario Downs, Emma Lawlor, Omar Martinez, Christina J. Sun, and Mary Claire O'Brien. 2015. "The Impact of Local Immigration Enforcement Policies on the Health of Immigrant Hispanics/Latinos in the United States." *American Journal of Public Health* 105 (2): 329–337.

Rice, Thomas. 2011. "UTMB Offers Patient Ticket to Mexico." *Houston Chronicle*, October 24, 2011.

Rice, Thomas, Pauline Rosenau, Lynn Y. Unruh, Andrew J. Barnes, Richard B. Saltman, Ewout van Ginneken. 2013. "United States of America: Health System Review." *Health Systems in Transition* 15 (3): 1–431.

Ridic, Goran, Suzanne Gleason, and Ognjen Ridic. 2012. "Comparisons of Health Care Systems in the United States, Germany and Canada." *Materia Socio-Medica* 24 (2): 112–120.

Ritzer, George. 2021. "McDonaldization in the Age of COVID-19." In *COVID-19: Global Pandemic, Societal Responses, Ideological Solutions*, edited by J. Michael Ryan, 23–28. New York: Routledge.

Romero, Mary. 2011. "Are Your Papers in Order: Racial Profiling, Vigilantes, and America's Toughest Sheriff." *Harvard Latino Law Review* 337: 345–352.

Rosenblum, Marc R., and Ariel G. Ruiz Soto. 2015. "An Analysis of Unauthorized Immigrants in the United States by Country and Region of Birth." Migration Policy Institute. www.migrationpolicy.org.

Salinas, Juan, and Manisha Salinas. 2022. "Systemic Racism and Undocumented Latino Migrant Laborers during COVID-19: A Narrative Review and Implications for Improving Occupational Health." *Journal of Migration and Health*, 5: 100106.

Sances, Michael, and Joshua D. Clinton. 2019. "Who Participated in the ACA? Gains in Insurance Coverage by Political Partisanship." *Journal of Health Politics, Policy and Law* 44 (3): 349–379.

Schaffer, Scott. 2021. "Necroethics in the Time of COVID-19 and Black Lives Matter." In *COVID-19: Global Pandemic, Societal Responses, Ideological Solutions*, edited by J. Michael Ryan, 43–53. New York: Routledge.

Schalk, Sami. 2017. "Critical Disability Studies as Methodology." *Lateral* 6 (1).

Schiff, Robert L., David A. Ansell, James E. Schlosser, Ahamed H. Idris, Ann Morrison, and Steven Whitman. 2019. "Transfers to a Public Hospital: A Prospective Study of 497 Patients." In *Community Health Equity: A Chicago Reader*, edited by Fernando De Maio, Raj C. Shah, John Mazzeo, and David A. Ansell, 226–237. Chicago: University of Chicago Press.

Schneider, Eric C., and David Squires. 2017. "From Last to First—Could the US Health Care System Become the Best in the World?" *New England Journal of Medicine* 377 (10): 901–903.

Seabury, Seth A., Sophie Terp, and Leslie I. Boden. 2017. "Racial and Ethnic Differences in the Frequency of Workplace Injuries and Prevalence of Work-Related Disability." *Health Affairs* 36 (2): 266–273.

Sears, Alan. 1999. "The 'Lean' State and Capitalist Restructuring: Towards a Theoretical Account." *Studies in Political Economy* 59 (1): 91–114.

Segers, Mary C. 1978. "Equality and Christian Anarchism: The Political and Social Ideas of the Catholic Worker Movement." *Review of Politics* 40 (2): 196–230.

Seim, Josh. 2017. "The Ambulance: Toward a Labor Theory of Poverty Governance." *American Sociological Review* 82 (3): 451–475.

Shakespeare, Tom. 2013. "The Social Model of Disability." In *The Disability Studies Reader*, 4th ed., edited by Lennard J. Davis, 214–221. New York: Routledge.

Shi, Leiyu, Jenna Tsai, Patricia Collins Higgins, and Lydie A. Lebrun. 2009. "Racial/Ethnic and Socioeconomic Disparities in Access to Care and Quality of Care for US Health Center Patients Compared with Non–Health Center Patients." *Journal of Ambulatory Care Management* 32 (4): 342–350.

Sirleaf, Matiangai V.S. 2021. "Disposable Lives: COVID-19, Vaccines, and the Uprising." *Columbia Law Review Forum* 121 (5): 71–94.

Small, Mario Luis. 2009. *Unanticipated Gains: Origins of Network Inequality in Everyday Life*. Oxford: Oxford University Press.

Smith, David E. 1976. "The Free Clinic Movement in the United States: A Ten Year Perspective (1966–1976)." *Journal of Drug Issues* 6 (4): 343–355.

Smith, David E., and Richard B. Seymour. 1997. "Addiction Medicine and the Free Clinic Movement." *Journal of Psychoactive Drugs* 29 (2): 155–160.

Smith, Michael D., and Dennis Wesselbaum. 2020. "COVID-19, Food Insecurity, and Migration." *Journal of Nutrition* 150 (11): 2855–2858.

Smith-Carrier, Tracy. 2020. "Charity Isn't Just, or Always Charitable: Exploring Charitable and Justice Models of Social Support." *Journal of Human Rights and Social Work* 5 (3): 157–163.

Soss, Joe, Richard C. Fording, and Sanford F. Schram. 2011. *Disciplining the Poor: Neoliberal Paternalism and the Persistent Power of Race.* Chicago: University of Chicago Press.

Spade, Dean. 2020a. *Mutual Aid: Building Solidarity during This Crisis (and the Next).* Brooklyn, NY: Verso Books.

———. 2020b. "Solidarity Not Charity: Mutual Aid for Mobilization and Survival." *Social Text* 38 (1): 131–151.

Stacker. 2022. "Biggest Sources of Immigrants to Phoenix." *Arizona's Family*, May 29, 2022. www.azfamily.com.

Staiti, Andrea B., Robert E. Hurley, and Aaron Katz. 2006. "Stretching the Safety Net to Serve Undocumented Immigrants: Community Responses to Health Needs." *Issue Brief (Center for Studying Health System Change)* 104 (1): 1–4.

Star, Susan Leigh. 1999. "The Ethnography of Infrastructure." *American Behavioral Scientist* 43 (3): 377–391.

Starfield, Barbara, Neil Powe, Jonathan R. Weiner, Mary Stuart, Donald Steinwachs, Sarah H. Scholle, and Andrea Gerstenberger. 1994. "Costs vs. Quality in Different Types of Primary Care Settings." *JAMA* 272 (24): 1903–1908.

Starr, Paul. 1982. "The Social Transformation of American Medicine." PhD diss., Harvard University.

State of Arizona Office of the Auditor General. 2009. "Maricopa County Special Health Care District: A Special Audit—Report to the Arizona State Legislature." www.azauditor.gov.

Stock, Paul V. 2014. "The Perennial Nature of the Catholic Worker Farms: A Reconsideration of Failure." *Rural Sociology* 79 (2): 143–173.

Stone, Robyn I. 2001. "Providing Long-Term Care Benefits in Cash: Moving to a Disability Model." *Health Affairs* 20 (6): 96–108.

Stovel, Katherine, Benjamin Golub, and Eva M. Meyersson Milgrom. 2011. "Stabilizing Brokerage." *Proceedings of the National Academy of Sciences* 108 (Supplement 4): 21326–21332.

Stovel, Katherine, and Lynette Shaw. 2012. "Brokerage." *Annual Review of Sociology* 38: 139–158.

Sutton, Janet, Raynard Washington, Kathryn Fingar, and Anne Elixhauser. 2016. "Characteristics of Safety-Net Hospitals, 2014." Statistical Brief #213. Healthcare Cost and Utilization Project. Agency for Healthcare Research and Quality (AHRQ). https://hcup-us.ahrq.gov.

Takeuchi, David T. 2016. "Vintage Wine in New Bottles: Infusing Select Ideas into the Study of Immigration, Immigrants, and Mental Health." *Journal of Health and Social Behavior* 57 (4): 423–435.

Takeuchi, David T., and Sue-Je L. Gage. 2003. "What to Do with Race? Changing Notions of Race in the Social Sciences." *Culture, Medicine and Psychiatry* 27 (4): 435–445.

Taylor, Rosemary CR. 1979. "Alternative Services: The Case of Free Clinics." *International Journal of Health Services* 9 (2): 227–253.

Tesler, Michael. 2012. "The Spillover of Racialization into Health Care: How President Obama Polarized Public Opinion by Racial Attitudes and Race." *American Journal of Political Science* 56 (3): 690–704.

Ticktin, Miriam. 2021. "Building a Feminist Commons in the Time of COVID-19." *Signs* 47 (1): 37–46.

Tikkanen, Roosa, Robin Osborn, Elias Mossialos, Ana Djordjevic, and George A. Wharton. 2020. "International Health Care System Profiles: United States." www.commonwealthfund.org.

Tolentino, Jia. 2020. "What Mutual Aid Can Do during a Pandemic." *New Yorker*, May 18, 2020. www.newyorker.com.

United States Census Bureau 2021. "Quickfact: Rochester City, New York." www.census.gov.

US Citizenship and Immigration Services (USCIS). 2009. "Public Charge." www.uscis.gov.

Van Natta, Meredith. 2019. "First Do No Harm: Medical Legal Violence and Immigrant Health in Coral County, USA." *Social Science & Medicine* 235: 112411.

———. 2023. *Medical Legal Violence: Health Care and Immigration Enforcement Against Latinx Noncitizens*. New York: NYU Press.

Van Natta, Meredith, Nancy J. Burke, Irene H. Yen, Mark D. Fleming, Christoph L. Hanssmann, Maryani Palupy Rasidjan, and Janet K. Shim. 2019. "Stratified Citizenship, Stratified Health: Examining Latinx Legal Status in the US Healthcare Safety Net." *Social Science & Medicine* 220: 49–55.

Varsanyi, Monica W., Paul G. Lewis, Doris Marie Provine, and Scott Decker. 2012. "A Multilayered Jurisdictional Patchwork: Immigration Federalism in the United States." *Law & Policy* 34 (2): 138–158.

Vernice, Nicholas A., Nicola M. Pereira, Anson Wang, Michelle Demetres, and Lisa V. Adams. 2020. "The Adverse Health Effects of Punitive Immigrant Policies in the United States: A Systematic Review." *PLoS ONE* 15 (12).

Viladrich, Anahí. 2005. "Tango Immigrants in New York City: The Value of Social Reciprocities." *Journal of Contemporary Ethnography* 34 (5): 533–559.

———. 2012. "Beyond Welfare Reform: Reframing Undocumented Immigrants' Entitlement to Health Care in the United States, a Critical Review." *Social Science & Medicine* 74 (6): 822–829.

Viruell-Fuentes, Edna A., Patricia Y. Miranda, and Sawsan Abdulrahim. 2012. "More than Culture: Structural Racism, Intersectionality Theory, and Immigrant Health." *Social Science & Medicine* 75 (12): 2099–2106.

Wacquant, Loïc. 2009. *Punishing the Poor: The Neoliberal Government of Social Insecurity.* Durham, NC: Duke University Press.

Waitzkin, Howard. 2000. *The Second Sickness: Contradictions of Capitalist Health Care.* 2nd ed. Lanham, MD: Rowman and Littlefield.

———. 2005. "Commentary—The History and Contradictions of the Health Care Safety Net." *Health Services Research* 40 (3): 941–952.

Waitzkin, Howard, and Rebeca Jasso-Aguilar. 2015. "Empire, Health, and Health Care: Perspectives at the End of Empire as We Have Known It." *Annual Review of Sociology* 41 (1): 271–290.

Wallace, Steven P., Jacqueline M. Torres, Tabashir Z. Nobari, and Nadereh Pourat. 2013. "Undocumented and Uninsured: Barriers to Affordable Care for Immigrant Populations." UCLA Center for Health Care Policy Research. https://escholarship.org/uc/item/8ds5h7k3.

Watson, Sidney D. 2009. "From Almshouses to Nursing Homes and Community Care: Lessons from Medicaid's History." *Georgia State University Law Review* 26: 937.

Watson, Tara. 2014. "Inside the Refrigerator: Immigration Enforcement and Chilling Effects in Medicaid Participation." *American Economic Journal: Economic Policy* 6 (3): 313–338.

Weber, Max. 1948. "Bureaucracy." In *Max Weber: Essays in Sociology*, 196–244. Abingdon, VA: Routledge.

Wells, Katie. 2021. "ERs Are Now Swamped with Seriously Ill Patients—but Many Don't Even Have COVID." National Public Radio. www.npr.org.

Wendell, Susan. 2013. "Unhealthy Disabled: Treating Chronic Illnesses as Disabilities." In *The Disability Studies Reader*, 4th ed., edited by Lennard J. Davis, 161–173. New York: Routledge.

Wetzstein, Steffen. 2017. "The Global Urban Housing Affordability Crisis." *Urban Studies* 54 (14): 3159–3177.

White, Kathryn V. 2017. "The Fiscal Survey of States." National Association of State Budget Officers. www.nasbo.org.

Wiener, Joshua M. 2013. "After CLASS: The Long-Term Care Commission's Search for a Solution." *Health Affairs* 32 (5): 831–834.

Williams, David R. 1999. "Race, Socioeconomic Status, and Health. The Added Effects of Racism and Discrimination." *Annals of the New York Academy of Sciences* 896: 173–188.

Williams, Vanessa. 2017. "'You Feel Invisible': How America's Fastest-Growing Immigrant Group Is Being Left out of the DACA Conversation." *Washington Post*, September 8, 2017.

Workers Defense Project. 2013. *Build a Better Texas.* Workers Defense Project. http://workersdefense.org.

Ye, Wei, and Javier M. Rodriguez. 2021. "Highly Vulnerable Communities and the Affordable Care Act: Health Insurance Coverage Effects, 2010–2018." *Social Science & Medicine* 270: 1–10.

Yudell, Michael, Dorothy Roberts, Rob DeSalle, Sarah Tishkoff, and 70 signatories. 2020. "NIH Must Confront the Use of Race in Science." *Science* 369 (6509): 1313–1314.

Zwick, Mark, and Louise Zwick. 2005. *The Catholic Worker Movement: Intellectual and Spiritual Origins*. New York: Paulist Press.

INDEX

Page numbers in *italics* indicate Figures

ABOUT THE AUTHORS

LISA SUN-HEE PARK is Professor of Asian American Studies at the University of California, Santa Barbara. Park's interdisciplinary research focuses on health care, migration, and environmental justice. She is the author of four other books, including *Entitled to Nothing: The Struggle for Immigrant Health Care in the Age of Welfare Reform*; *The Slums of Aspen: Immigrants vs. the Environment in America's Eden* (co-authored with David N. Pellow), which received the Outstanding Book Award from the American Sociological Association's Environment and Technology Section; and *Consuming Citizenship: Children of Asian Immigrant Entrepreneurs*, which received the Outstanding Book Award from the American Sociological Association's Asia and Asian America Section.

ERIN HOEKSTRA is an independent scholar. She was Assistant Professor of Sociology in the Department of Social and Cultural Sciences at Marquette University. Her research and activism focus on immigration and health justice in the US-Mexico borderlands. Her work has been published in *Social Science & Medicine* and the *Journal of Ethnic & Migration Studies*.

ANTHONY M. JIMENEZ is Assistant Professor of Sociology at the Rochester Institute of Technology. Born and raised in El Paso, Texas, along the US-Mexico border, Jimenez centers his interdisciplinary research on border imperialism and intersections between immigration and health care. His work has been supported by the Ford Foundation and appears in journals such as *Social Science & Medicine*, the *Journal of Ethnic & Migration Studies*, and the *Journal of Immigrant and Minority Health*.

Printed in the United States
by Baker & Taylor Publisher Services